KU-647-671

HEALTH OF THE NATION: THE BMJ VIEW

Edited by

RICHARD SMITH, MD

Editor, British Medical Journal

Articles from the *British Medical Journal*

Published by the British Medical Journal
Tavistock Square, London WC1H 9JR

© British Medical Journal 1991

All rights reserved. No part of this publication may be reproduced, stored in a retrieval system, or transmitted, in any form or by any means, electronic, mechanical, photocopying, recording and/or otherwise, without the prior written permission of the publishers.

First published 1991

British Library Cataloguing in Publication Data

Health of the Nation.

ISBN 0–7279–0314–4

The following picture sources are acknowledged:

Front cover, ADT London Marathon 1991 courtesy of ADT; page 13, Ian Showell/Press Association; page 32, Judy Harrison/Format; page 38, Brenda Prince; page 52 John K Simmons; page 66, John Rae; page 78, Bill Aron/Science Library; pages 151 and 201, Mark Edwards/ Still Pictures; pages 158 and 164, Sally and Richard Greenhill; page 212, Lorraine Jones/Format; page 216, Chris Priest, Mark Clarke/Science Photo Library.

Typeset by Bedford Typesetters Limited, Bedford
Printed and bound in Great Britain by
Latimer Trend & Company Ltd, Plymouth

Contents

HAROLD BRIDGES LIBRARY
S. MARTIN'S COLLEGE
LANCASTER

First steps towards a strategy for health

RICHARD SMITH

We are clear about one thing: a strategy imposed by government which takes no heed of the views of those who will have to implement it, including the people themselves, is valueless.

This quote from Mr William Waldegrave, Secretary of State for Health comes from his introduction to *The Health of the Nation*, the consultative document that sets out a strategy for improving the health of the English.[1] It's a pity that the strategy for the NHS didn't follow the same philosophy (and Mr Waldegrave has said so himself),[2] but it is true that the strategy for health will not work if the many individuals and organisations that will have to act to make it work do not feel any ownership. As John Harvey-Jones, the former chief executive officer of ICI, explains in his book *Making it Happen*, this does not have to mean that the strategy degenerates to the lowest common denominator that everyone can agree on: people and organisations will put their backs into making a strategy work as long as they are convinced that they have been heard—even if not all of their proposals have been accepted.[3] And they cannot all be. As Mr Waldegrave says elsewhere in his introduction: "priorities are meaningless if they include everything."

Taking Mr Waldegrave at his word on wanting to listen to everybody, this book comprises a response to *The Health of the Nation*. The chapters address each of the 16 key areas identified in the strategy and other subjects that might qualify as key areas. For each key area the authors have been asked to make the case that it should be a key area; consider the case against; identify what the targets should be within the key area; suggest a strategy for reaching the targets; and then identify barriers to reaching them. Not all of the chapters follow exactly this format.

1

Why a strategy?

Effective organisations know where they are going. "The secret of success," said Benjamin Disraeli, "is constancy to purpose." Organisations that drift—like much of British industry in the past—are prone to disappear. Organisations that have strategies can concentrate on what they do best and devote resources (which are always limited) accordingly. The strategy should motivate people and allow them to work hardest at the activities that will produce the richest return. Setting a strategy also forces people to look to the future, making it more likely that they will see emerging opportunities early and be able to exploit them and notice the spot on the horizon that is an express train coming to destroy them—giving them a chance to get out of the way.

The figure is a device for analysing the effectiveness of organisations. The more effective live in the top right hand corner and have a clear vision that is shared by most of those within the organisation: Toyota, IBM, Sainsbury's, the Vietcong, and Intenational Physicians for the Prevention of Nuclear War have been in this square. Most organisations exist in the least effective, bottom left hand corner—with little sense of collective vision. The NHS has probably been in the bottom right hand corner with a vision that has been shared but unclear. *The Health of the Nation* might push it to the effective top right hand corner, or disagreements and poor morale within the service might push it into the bottom left hand corner, where even the sense of working together on something important is lost. The next few years will tell.

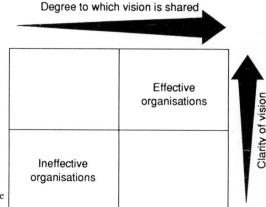

Effective and ineffective organisations

The Department of Health has come late to the idea of a strategy with targets.[4 5] The World Health Organisation set targets in 1978 with its slogan of "health for all by the year 2000"[6] and the European Office of WHO followed this up with its 38 targets in 1985.[7] The United States,[8] Wales,[9] Scotland,[10] Northern Ireland,[11] and many other countries[4] have all set targets during a time when the English Department of Health seemed sniffy about the whole process. Why, cynics inevitably wonder, has the department come round? Is it a change of minister or, as *The Health of the Nation* suggests, because the reforming of the NHS has made possible what was previously impossible? Or is it to divert political attention from the agonies of the NHS? Whatever the reason the strategy deserves to be taken at face value.

What sort of strategy?

Once an organisation has decided that it needs a strategy there are various ways to go about developing it. Essentially the organisation must make a detailed analysis of its present position (and the professors of strategy have many ways to cut the cake); then it must decide where it wants to go and how it is going to get there. The Department of Health has many difficulties with this process: the data for fully assessing the present position are, as *The Health of the Nation* concedes, inadequate; it is politically difficult for the department to draw up a full list of weaknesses and strengths in the way that a company would do behind closed doors; and the strategy is not just for one organisation but for many. The glossy document is disappointingly repetitive and defensive, and there is much more on the NHS than on the broader aspects of health.

The Department of Health has defined the aim of the strategy—"to improve the span of healthy life"—and then combined this aim with some "key strategic policy objectives and guiding principles." These comprise focusing on the "main health problems"; concentrating as much on promotion of health as on treatment, care, and rehabilitation (but without setting up a false conflict between either); recognising that the health services are only one influence on health; encouraging greater cooperation between those inside and outside the NHS; combining central strategic direction with "local and individual direction, flexibility, and initiative"; and securing the best use of resources.

3

Possible key areas

Causes of substantial mortality
- Coronary heart disease
- Stroke
- Cancers
- Accidents

Causes of substantial ill health
- Mental health
- Diabetes
- Asthma

Contributing factors to both mortality and morbidity and to healthy living
- Smoking
- Diet and alcohol
- Physical exercise

Where there is clear scope for improvement
- Health of pregnant women, infants, and children
- Rehabilitation services for people with a physical disability
- Environmental quality

Where there is a great potential for harm
- HIV and AIDS
- Other communicable diseases
- Food safety

Following these guidelines the department has then begun to identify "key areas." There are three criteria for a subject becoming a key area: it should be a major cause of premature death or avoidable ill health; interventions offering "significant scope for improvement in health" must be available; and it must be possible to set targets within the key area and then monitor them. The box shows candidate key areas identified in the strategy.

Within each key area targets are to be set that are "realistic but challenging." They are "so far as is possible [to] be expressed in terms of health improvements or—where appropriate—reductions in risk factors. . . or precursors of ill health." "Above all," says the strategy, "objectives and targets should be agreed by all those who have a part to play in their achievement." Other criteria might have been used, and the Faculty of Public Health Medicine has recently emphasised the criteria used by McGinnis (box).[12][13]

Most health strategies revolve around measurable targets, and most would agree that this is wholly right. There are, however, problems with targets, as the Faculty of Public Health Medicine has emphasised in its report published in the summer of 1991 on levels of health in the United Kingdom.[12] Firstly, they may lead to spurious priority being given to that which is measurable. Secondly, they may represent an oversimplistic description of policy. Thirdly, they may appear unrealistic and be easily dismissed as unattainable.

There may also be practical problems in setting a target. Thus some have used computer modelling, but the government seems to have largely plucked its targets out of the sky. They are the product of "informed judgment," or guesswork.

Making it happen

The easy part of strategic planning is devising a strategy. The

---

Criteria for indicators and targets

Indicators and targets should be:

- *Credible*—Address important public health issues that are likely to remain current
- *Clear*—Easily appraised by and relevant to a wide general audience
- *Selective*—The choice of topic should be used to highlight areas that are a high priority for action
- *Compatible*—With current public health strategies
- *Achievable*—Interventions should be available or potentially available. The target must take account of evidence of effectiveness and the delay between intervention and effect
- *Balanced*—Monitor progress through a mixture of process and outcome measures
- *Quantifiable*—Data for the whole United Kingdom are required; if necessary proxy indicators should be used or specific recommendations made for the collection of data
- *Ethical*—Respect the autonomy of individuals and avoid unnecessary value judgments

---

Those with a role in implementing the strategy

- Individuals
- Families
- Communities
- Health care services
- Personal social services
- Health professions
- The education service
- Voluntary sector
- Industry, commerce, and trades unions
- The media
- Government—central and local
- International organisations

---

difficult part is making it happen. And this is especially true when so many groups are potentially involved. The last box lists some of those who may have a part to play in implementing England's health strategy. The Department of Health is inviting comments from anybody interested and plans after consultation to "issue a further document which will define and set in motion a health strategy for England."

Some governments have set targets and then left it to others to work out how to achieve them. The Department of Health insists that it will be more hands on, but at the same time it doesn't want to stifle "local discretion." Thus the secretary of state has set up an "English Health Strategy Steering Group" to advise him. It will be supported by three expert working groups: one to cover "the wider public and political dimensions" and link industry, the media, and other government departments; one to consider health priorities and measure progress and develop scientific interventions; and one to look at how the NHS can implement the strategy.

Within the NHS the secretary of state can at least crack the whip and make sure that the strategy is "built into NHS management systems—contracts, collaborative arrangements, audit, planning, monitoring and review." The green paper spells out what regional and district health authorities, family health services authorities, and provider units might do.

For the health strategy to have real impact the other groups who may have a part to play in implementing the strategy will also have to take action, especially as the health services themselves have only a limited impact on health. And why should Thames Television, Nuneaton Social Services, or the BMA do their bit for the health strategy? They will have to be persuaded, which is why real consultation is so important. And most difficult of all to persuade might be other government departments. The Department of Health is way down the Cabinet pecking order, and why should the Treasury reduce its income from tobacco, or the Department of Trade and Industry give up on its plans to promote the alcohol industry, one of Britain's biggest exporters and employers? But if the government is at all serious about health then these big fish must be encouraged to swim with the strategy otherwise the many small fish will be reluctant to contribute.

The next problem after initial implementation is to sustain motivation and commitment. This is a particular problem with politically driven strategies—because another party coming to power may be unwilling to follow its opponent's strategy or indeed any strategy.

Conclusion

Many of the contributors to this book are critical of aspects of the government's strategy, but almost all of them support the idea of a strategy. The government should welcome vigorous debate of its proposals because that is the only way to arrive at a robust strategy to which everybody will be keen to contribute.

1 Secretary of State for Health. *The Health of the Nation*. London: HMSO, 1991.
2 Smith R. William Waldegrave: thinking on the new NHS. *BMJ* 1991;**302**:636-40.
3 Harvey-Jones J. *Making it happen*. Glasgow: Collins, 1988.
4 Catford JC. Health targets. *BMJ* 1991;**302**:980-1.
5 Ashton J. The health of the nation. *BMJ* 1991;**302**:1413-4.
6 World Health Organisation. *Alma Ata 1978. Primary health care*. Geneva: WHO, 1978.
7 World Health Organisation Regional Office for Europe. *Targets for health for all*. Copenhagen: WHO, 1985.
8 US Public Health Service. *Healthy people. Surgeon General's report on health promotion and disease prevention*. Washington, DC: US Department of Health and Human Services, 1979.
9 Health Promotion Authority for Wales. *Health for all in Wales: health promotion challenges for the 1990s*. Cardiff: Health Promotion Authority for Wales, 1990.

10 Scottish Office Home and Health Department. *Health education in Scotland—a national policy statement*. Edinburgh: HMSO, 1991.

11 Northern Ireland Health Promotion Agency. *Health promotion in Northern Ireland. A discussion paper*. Belfast: Northern Ireland Health Promotion Agency, 1990.

12 The Faculty of Public Health Medicine of the Royal College of Physicians. *UK levels of health*. London: Faculty of Public Health Medicine, 1991.

13 McGinnis JM. Setting objectives for public health in the 1990s: experience and prospects. *Annu Rev Public Health* 1990;**11**:231-49.

Missing: a strategy for the health of the nation

RADICAL STATISTICS HEALTH GROUP

In 1978 the World Health Organisation took the lead towards a clearly defined and quantifiable global strategy for promoting health.[1-3] Through Health for All by the Year 2000 the WHO called on each of its regions to identify appropriate targets for health to be achieved by the year 2000.[4 5] The United Kingdom government was a formal signatory but has consistently failed to endorse the 38 targets for health identified by WHO's European region[6] despite the fact that over 70 local authorities and health authorities in England have independently adopted the European strategy.[7]

Now, after a decade of resistance, does the publication of the green paper *The Health of the Nation* mark a change in policy?[8] We have serious reservations. Although the government has monitored its progress towards WHO's targets,[9] it seems to have rejected many of them and is now setting its own. The targets it proposes seem to be restricted by two concerns: to maximise the efficiency or output of the NHS and to change the behaviour of individuals. Absent from the paper are three principles that are central to the WHO strategy. These are the philosophy that all government policies should take into account their impact on the health of the population, the need to redress social inequalities, and the importance of community participation. The WHO considers that these principles are essential for any strategy to have a successful impact on the health of the nation.[1]

Why now?

The renewed political interest in targets dates back to October 1990 when Kenneth Clarke, then Secretary of State for Health, announced the intention of developing a portfolio of targets for health care. His

9

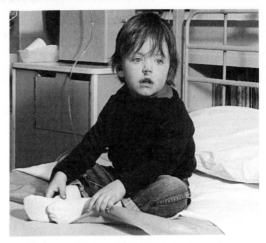

Lack of morbidity data on children and others means targets are performance related

view was that targets give those in the NHS a tangible objective to aim at and provide a way of measuring success and evaluating what we are getting for our investment in the NHS. (Department of Health press release, October 1990 (90/1487)). The impression given was of targets that had less to do with health than with the business management ethos of *Working for Patients*.[10]

The government's embarrassment over the difficulties caused by the changes to the NHS must have made the idea of announcing a national strategy for health attractive. In the event a curious and muddled collection of targets has emerged. Some targets relate to efficiency in the NHS, some to disease prevention, some to health promotion, and others to quality of service. The lack of a unifying framework reflects the absence of overall strategy and of relevant data to implement and monitor it. In view of the way the green paper has emerged great care is needed to look beneath the superficial gloss of this document and to question its likely impact on the health of the nation. Several areas of concern emerge.

A strategy for health?

The first problem is that the document confuses a strategy for health with a strategy for the health service. Furthermore, most of the initiatives are not even new. For example, projects cited include Look After Your Heart, the smoking programme, the Joint Breast Feeding Initiative, the workplace scheme, and cervical and breast cancer screening.[11 12]

All these programmes overemphasise individual responsibility without sufficiently considering the barriers which make it difficult for some people to change their lifestyle. For example, the strategy for dealing with alcohol related diseases is confined to exhortations to keep "within the sensible drinking limits." The document states that "smoking during pregnancy is associated with low birthweight babies and also a 28% increase in perinatal mortality in babies." The proposed strategy is to "provide information and support to women to enable them to stop smoking during pregnancy" with a grant of £1 million to the Health Education Authority. This ignores the evidence that socioeconomic factors not only contribute to the likelihood of women smoking but operate independently to increase the risk of having a low birthweight baby.[13] Socioeconomic factors also influence smoking among adults more generally: members of the manual classes are more likely to smoke than those in non-manual classes, but no attempt is made to target this disparity. Though the document recognises that the prevention of alcohol and smoking related diseases is sensitive to both legislation and pricing,[14] it contains no specific proposals for legal and fiscal measures.

For road traffic accidents, which caused 4938 deaths in England and Wales in 1989,[15] and in which there are appreciable social class differences[16] the approach is to increase public awareness rather than to develop policies and enforce measures related to safety. Other types of accidents are mentioned but no preventive measures are proposed.

A further limitation of the green paper is its focus on particular diseases and habits instead of on the groups within the population and their problems. As a result, many of the targets relate to the treatment of disease rather than the promotion of health. Though targets are set for reducing mortality from ischaemic heart disease and stroke, there is also a health care performance target for ischaemic heart disease, based on the number of coronary artery bypass grafts operations per million population.

In the discussion of asthma, a disease in which the incidence is rising, there is no mention of the aetiology of asthma or its association with bad housing conditions and damp.[17] Instead of setting targets for reducing the incidence of asthma, indicators of clinical practice are chosen, with a recommendation that the outcome measures should reflect "adherence to published clinical management guidelines."

Where groups within the population are considered the emphasis is on setting narrow "medical" targets. Disability is an example of an area where multisectoral influences are more important than medical services alone. The barriers to integration with the rest of society include poverty, legislation, segregated education, lack of accessible buildings, transport, employment prospects, and personal assistance.[18-20]

The green paper not only seems to ignore the vast amount of work on person based outcome measures relating to disability[21-25] but fails to give prominence to the third WHO target: "By the year 2000, disabled people should have the physical, social and economic opportunities that allow at least for a socially and economically fulfilling and mentally creative life." Instead, the stated objective is "to enable people with physical disabilities to reach an optimal level of *functioning*" and suggested targets are confined to reducing contractures and incontinence and pressure sores by 5-10%. Policies and targets recognising the need for multisectoral change across departments and coordinated legislation are completely absent.

Health promotion activities pursued solely within the NHS are unlikely to improve the nation's health. Concerted action is needed from many government departments with policies to reduce homelessness, increase income support, protect the environment including reduction of air and water pollution, improve public transport, and promote health and safety at work. Fiscal and legal measures are needed to discourage consumption of alcohol and tobacco and to make food safe. Above all policies are needed to reverse the growing inequalities in health in our society. All these are vital components for a national programme aimed at enhancing the nation's health and all are absent from *The Health of the Nation*. Only six of its 151 pages are explicitly devoted to action outside the NHS, and these merely contain lists of central government departments and their activities. Thus, while citing a century of achievements in housing and describing improvements since the 1960s it contains little indication of the new policies and initiatives required to combat the adverse impact on health of a decade of escalating homelessness and substandard housing.[26-28]

Measurement problems

As measurability is a criterion the choice of targets is constrained by the availability of relevant information. It is not surprising that lack of information itself is not worth targeting. The lack of morbidity data needed to measure and monitor the health of the population and subsections within it is a well known and longstanding problem.[29-31]

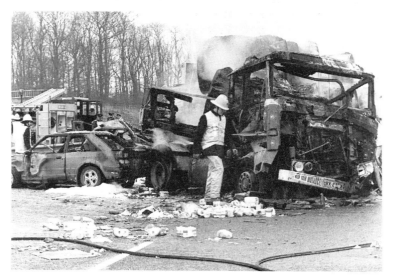

Increased public awareness not safety measures is relied on to reduce road traffic accidents

As usual, the authors of the document are left dependent on mortality and activity statistics. For example, there are few routine data on the prevalence of ill health and disability among elderly people, children, people with disabilities and mental illness, and those in need of terminal care or rehabilitation. This makes it difficult to set reductions in morbidity as targets and so instead targets have been chosen that relate to performance such as reducing bed occupancy and closing psychiatric hospitals. In the absence of morbidity data, alternative targets could have related to aspects of care, such as implementing care in the community[32] by improving the availability and range of community and domiciliary services.

Food poisoning and HIV infection have been excluded from target setting on the grounds that information on cause and incidence is inadequate. The government seems reluctant to develop strategies to tackle these infections, although a great deal is known about their aetiology and their mode of transmission.

Methodological problems are also ignored. There is no systematic analysis of past and projected trends in the indicators chosen. Such an analysis would need to consider whether these trends reflect changes in clinical practice, health promotion, lifestyles, the age structure of

13

the population, or the many socioeconomic factors that can affect health. For example, no attempt is made to interpret the fall in smoking prevalence, the decline in mortality from ischaemic heart disease and stroke, or changes in asthma incidence.

Other statistical questions are those associated with random variation. For example regional and district health authorities are asked to set targets for stillbirth rates and infant mortality, but the small number of deaths in each district means that rates are subject to wide random variations from year to year.[33]

Inequalities in health

The first of the WHO's targets for the European region is: "By the year 2000, the actual differences in health status between countries and between groups within countries should be reduced by at least 25%, by improving the levels of health of disadvantaged nations and groups." This is dismissed as being "unlikely on present evidence to be achieved." In doing so, the green paper ignores a wealth of detailed evidence on inequalities,[34-36] thereby sidestepping the need for action. This rejection is in line with the philosophy of *Working for Patients*,[10] which turns its back on the original aim of the NHS — equality in both health and access to health care.[37]

Countries that have developed strategies for achieving targets for health have equity as a main criterion for selecting priorities in line with the first WHO target.[38] Though there are methodological problems in comparing inequalities in health in different countries, but it is apparent that inequalities in health, as measured by morbidity and mortality, are wider in England and Wales than in Sweden.[39 40] In addition, the gap is not widening in many countries as it is in England and Wales.[41 42] Thus inequalities in health are not inevitable even if no society is free of them.

Widening differentials in wealth in the United Kingdom might be expected to be followed by corresponding inequalities in health. Internationally there is a crude relation between the magnitude of inequalities in income and magnitude of inequalities in health.[42] Overall life expectancy is lower in countries with wide income differentials independent of gross national product.[43] There is no evidence that simply relying on an increase in the overall wealth will reduce the numbers of people in poverty or diminish the gap in health.[44 45]

In the absence of both a criterion stipulating equity and the necessary data to monitor it the needs of people who are not well placed to respond to health promotion and health care initiatives may be neglected in favour of those who are better able to do so. Thus health promotion initiatives may target those in the population who can make a larger contribution to "health care" as measured by health statistics. This could result in an inverse health law to parallel Julian Tudor Hart's inverse care law that the availability of good medical care tends to vary inversely with the need for it in the population served.[46]

Views of the public

Where does the public fit into all this? The views of the public are mentioned only once in the entire document and then only in the context of family health services authorities. Surveys of people's attitudes to restricting smoking in public places and increasing taxation show that most would support these measures.[47 48] A Health Education Authority survey showing that pollution and the environment were perceived by the public as the major threats to health[49] was cited in an earlier draft of the green paper as an indication of how badly people were informed. These are just two examples of government disregard for public opinion.

Implementing the strategy

The document states that the government will not only set up the strategy but take an active role in its implementation through the English National Strategy Steering Group, which will be supported by three expert working panels. The constitution of these groups and, more importantly, the power they will have in reaching the targets are not mentioned. Will other departments be represented and forced to follow decisions made by these groups? How will districts and people at the grass roots be represented? Though some have praised the document for making government accountable, an alternative scenario, not dissimilar to that of local authority expenditure, is that ineffective management will be used as a scapegoat in poor districts that fail to achieve the necessary reductions.

It must not be forgotten that the changes in the NHS were introduced in part to distract attention from the underfunding of the NHS. The strategy proposes that as much emphasis should be placed on the promotion of health as on the treatment of ill health, but gives

15

no commitment to extra resources. Under such conditions, will the strategy have a detrimental effect on access to health care by people who are already ill? In a cost contained NHS how will health authorities choose between health promotion and health care? Will they be forced to invest in ineffectual health promotion policies in the mistaken belief that these will promote health? What sections of the community will benefit from this shift in resources? Will resources be shifted away from health care for elderly, poor, and disabled people to fund health education campaigns for the younger, healthier, and more affluent people, who are able to respond to campaigns to change their behaviour? Or will little more be done in health promotion because no funds are being made available and the targets identified will probably be achieved through existing programmes?

Conclusion

The scope for improving health largely lies outside the NHS, but the key role of the NHS as a service to provide treatment, care, and rehabilitation must be safeguarded in a revised strategy. If the NHS persists in trying to tackle health single handed it will be held accountable for making promises it cannot keep. Worse still it will be distracted into forgetting the groups in the population whose needs are being ignored in the arguments about efficiency, health gains, and health benefits.

An effective strategy for the nation's health must therefore distinguish what the health service can achieve in both providing health care and promoting health and then set out clearly the responsibility of other government departments and agencies for promoting health in a wider sense. It needs to collect the data required to implement and monitor strategies rather than opportunistically shape strategy to the restrictions of existing data. Above all, there must be commitment to reducing inequalities in health and to providing the resources and mechanisms needed for implementing strategies successfully.

1 World Health Organisation. *Alma Ata 1978. Primary health care.* Geneva: WHO, 1978. (Health for all series No 1.)
2 World Health Organisation. *Global strategy for health by the year 2000.* Geneva: WHO, 1981. (Health for all series No 3.)
3 World Health Organisation. *Development of indicators for monitoring progress towards health for all by the year 2000.* Geneva: WHO, 1981.
4 World Health Organisation Regional Office for Europe. *Targets for health for all.* Copenhagen: WHO, 1985.

5 World Health Organisation Regional Office for Europe. *European regional strategy for attaining health for all.* Copenhagen: WHO, 1981. (EUR/RC 30/8 Rev 2.)

6 *The United Kingdom monitoring report on the strategy for Health for All by the year 2000, 1985-1988.* London: Department of Health. International Division.

7 United Kingdom health for all. *Network News* Spring/Summer 1991.

8 Department of Health. *The health of the nation: a consultative document for health in England.* London: HMSO, 1991. (Cm 1523.)

9 Department of Health. *On the state of the public health for the year 1989.* London: HMSO, 1990.

10 Secretaries of State for Health, Wales, Northern Ireland, and Scotland. *Working for Patients.* London: HMSO, 1989.

11 Health Education Authority. *Strategic plan 1990-95.* London: Health Education Authority, 1989.

12 Health Education Authority. *Heart disease in the 1990s. A strategy for 1990-95.* The Health Education Authority, Look after Your Heart programme. London.

13 Rush D, Cassano P. Relationship of cigarette smoking and social class to birth weight and perinatal mortality among all births in Britain, 5-11 April 1970. *J Epidemiol Community Health* 1983;**37**:249-55.

14 Godfrey C. Modelling demand. In: Maynard A, Tether P, eds. *Preventing alcohol and tobacco problems.* Vol 1. Avebury, 1990.

15 Office of Population Censuses and Surveys. *Mortality statistics, accidents and violence 1988.* London: HMSO, 1991. (Series DH14 No 15.)

16 Office of Population Censuses and Surveys. *Occupational mortality 1979-80, 1982-83, Great Britain. Decennial supplement.* London: HMSO, 1986. (Series DS No 6.)

17 Strachan DP. Damp, housing, mould allergy, and childhood asthma. *Proceedings of the Royal College of Physicians* 1991;**21**:140-6.

18 Bowe F. *Handicapping America.* New York: Harper and Rowe, 1978.

19 Gloag D. Unmet need in chronic disability. *BMJ* 1984;**289**:211-2.

20 Office of Population and Censuses and Surveys. *OPCS surveys of disability in Great Britain. Report 2: the financial circumstances of disabled adults living in private households.* London: HMSO, 1988.

21 Hirst M. Multidimensional representation of disablement. In: Baldwin S, Godfrey C, Propper C, eds. *Quality of life. Perspectives and policies.* London: Routledge, 1990.

22 Clark A, Hirst M. Disability in adulthood: ten year follow-up of young people with disabilities. *Disability, Handicap and Society* 1989;**4**:271-83.

23 Royal College of Physicians. *Health Service for adults with physical disabilities. A survey of district health authorities 1988/89.* London: RCP, 1990.

24 Gloag D. Needs and opportunities in rehabilitation. Severe disability. 2. Residential care and living in the community. *BMJ* 1985;**290**:368-72.

25 Gloag D. Needs and opportunities in rehabilitation. Introduction and a look at some short term orthopaedic rehabilitation. *BMJ* 1985;**290**:43-6.

26 Lowry S. *Housing and Health.* London: British Medical Journal, 1991.

27 Mant DC, Muir Gray JA. *Building regulations and health.* Watford: Building Research Establishment, 1986.

28 Connelly J, Kelleher C, Morton S, St George D, Roderick P, eds. *Housing or homelessness: a public health perspective.* London: Faculty of Public Health Medicine, 1991.

29 Thunhurst C, Macfarlane AJ. Monitoring the health of urban populations: what statistics do we need? *Journal of the Royal Statistical Society, Series A* (in press).

30 Macfarlane AJ, McPherson CK. The quality of official health statistics. *Journal of the Royal Statistical Society, Series A* 1988;**151**:342-54.

31 Radical Statistics Health Group. *The unofficial guide to official health statistics.* London: Radical Statistics, 1980.

32 Department of Health and Social Security. *Caring for people—community care in the next decade and beyond.* London: HMSO, 1989.

33 Macfarlane AJ, Mugford M. *Birth counts: statistics of pregnancy and childbirth.* London: HMSO, 1984.

34 Working Group on Inequalities in Health. *Inequalities in health.* London: Department of Health and Social Security, 1980.

35 Whitehead M. *The health divide in inequalities in health.* London: Penguin, 1988.

36 Research Unit in Health and Behavioural Change. *Changing the public health.* Chichester: John Wiley, 1989.

37 Ministry of Health, Department of Health for Scotland. *A National Health Service*. London: HMSO, 1944. (Cmnd 6502.)

38 Department of Health. *Operational research. Setting strategic health goals: experience in other countries. Report of a preliminary review*. London: DoH, 1990. (ORZ/1297.)

39 Lundberg O. Class and health: comparing Britain and Sweden. *Soc Sci Med* 1986:**23**:511-7.

40 Vagero D, Lundberg O. Health inequalities in Britain and Sweden. *Lancet* 1989;iii:35-6.

41 Marmot MG, McDowall M. Mortality decline and widening social inequalities. *Lancet* 1986;ii:274-6.

42 Davey Smith G, Bartley M, Blane D. The Black report on socioeconomic inequalities in health 10 years on. *BMJ* 1990;**301**:373-7.

43 Wilkinson RG. Income distribution and mortality: a natural experiment. *Sociology of Health and Illness* 1990;**12**:391-412.

44 Wilkinson RG. Class mortality differentials, income distribution and trends in social poverty 1921-1981. *Journal of Social Policy* 1989;**18**:307-35.

45 Mr Major's dream: is social mobility enough? *Lancet* 1990;**336**:1547-8.

46 Tudor Hart J. The inverse care law. *Lancet* 1971;i:405-12.

47 Health Education Authority. *Young peoples' health and lifestyles (Marketing and Opinion Research Institute poll*. London: Health Education Authority, 1989.

48 Health Education Authority. *Smoking habits (National Opinion Poll)*. London: Health Education Authority, 1989.

49 Health Education Authority. *National Opinion Poll consumer health education survey, 1987-1989*. London: Health Education Authority, 1990.

Dietary aspects of a health strategy for England

S BINGHAM

Diet has a key role in the prevention of the major life threatening conditions of middle and later life, especially cardiovascular disease and probably cancer. Its role in the aetiology of diabetes, osteoporosis, arthritis, inflammatory bowel disease, and dementia is also under investigation. The benefit of a correct diet in preventing constipation, obesity, and dental caries has been proved. All this is in addition to its classic roles in growth, maintaining normal physiological functions, and preventing deficiency diseases such as anaemia, rickets, and pellagra. In cardiovascular disease and cancer alone, conditions which account for over 60% of deaths in the United Kingdom, about 30% of attributable risk can probably be ascribed to diet.

With this substantial contribution to health and prevention of disease, it is not surprising that diet is a recurring theme throughout the recent green paper *The Health of the Nation*.[1] However, political acceptance of the potential for good health through food represents a remarkable change of emphasis that should have wide ranging consequences for agriculture, the food industry, advertising, food science, departments of public health, and ultimately the consumer.

The case for diet as a key target in the health strategy is easy to justify. Mortality from coronary heart disease in the United Kingdom is among the highest in the world, accounting for more deaths and more premature deaths than any other single cause. Though genetic variation in apolipoproteins is important in determining susceptibility to coronary heart disease, about half the risk is attributable to smoking, high blood pressure, and raised serum cholesterol concentrations, with the last two being profoundly affected by diet.

19

Hypertension, which is a risk factor for stroke, is related to alcohol consumption, obesity, high dietary sodium intake, and reduced intakes of potassium and possibly calcium and magnesium[2]; relative risk of stroke is increased fourfold in people with usual diastolic blood pressures of 105 mm Hg and above.[3]

Consumption of fatty acids

The effect of different saturated fatty acids on serum cholesterol concentrations and associated coronary heart disease risk is well established.[45] Genetic control means that there are substantial individual differences in serum cholesterol responses and this partly accounts for the low correlation between single estimates of diet and serum cholesterol measurements.[6] Other dietary factors associated with coronary heart disease include obesity, alcohol, and the protective effect of antioxidant vitamins, dietary fibre, and minerals. These may explain some anomalies in the epidemiology but do not negate the substantial case against saturated fats. Saturated fatty acids and dietary cholesterol suppress low density lipoprotein receptor activity, and controlled metabolic studies have repeatedly confirmed that they raise serum cholesterol concentrations.[2]

Sixty seven per cent of the variance in plasma cholesterol concentration is attributable to myristic acid (C14) which is found in dairy fats and meat, with palmitic acid (C16) having a lesser effect. There is no evidence that stearic acid (C18) or shorter chain saturated fatty acids (less than C14) raise serum cholesterol concentrations.[4] Another role for dietary fat is that of the $\omega3$ polyunsaturated fats (fish oils), which inhibit thromboxane A_3 and hence reduce blood clotting.[7] The role of monounsaturates (in olive oil) characteristic of the Mediterranean diet in the prevention of coronary heart disease and of stroke is less clear. Populations at low risk of coronary heart disease with a high intake of monounsaturated fatty acids also consume low amounts of saturated fatty acids.[3]

Given the weight of evidence that consumption of saturated fat is related to risk of coronary heart disease, how much should we be eating? The average serum cholesterol concentration in British adults is currently 5·8 mmol/l, and about two thirds of the population have concentrations above the desirable level of 5·2 mmol/l.[8] Average intake of saturated fatty acids is 36·5 g/day, or 16% of total dietary energy. The recently published dietary reference values recommend a reduction of saturated fat to 10% of total dietary energy,[4] which should result in an average lowering of cholesterol concentrations by 0·4 mmol/l to 5·4 mmol/l. A greater reduction in coronary heart disease will be achieved if these changes are confined to C14 and C16 fatty acids and if consumption of soluble non-starch polysaccharide (dietary fibre) is increased.[4]

The green paper targets are set in terms of population distributions for food energy (excluding alcohol) (table I) but are consistent with the average recommended dietary reference values. The ultimate goal of the green paper proposals is for a 30% reduction in premature deaths from coronary heart disease between 1988 and 2000, to be achieved partly by the above dietary change, together with a reduction in smoking, increased physical activity, and reduction in hypertension. If the reduction in saturated fat intake is achieved, the goal is theoretically achievable as the relation between serum cholesterol concentration and mortality from coronary heart disease alone predicts about a 20% fall in mortality with a reduction of serum cholesterol concentration from 5·8 to 5·4 mmol/l.[5]

Other targets

The second target is that at least 50% of the population should derive less than 35% of their food energy from total fat by the year 2005. This is equivalent to a population average for total fat

TABLE I—Government population distribution targets for food consumption and obesity related to present distributions, and present and recommended consumption of saturated and total fat

	Proportion of population (%)		Population average consumption as proportion of food energy (%)	
	Target distribution for 2005	Present distribution	Present	Dietary recommended value[4]
Derive <15% food energy from saturated fat	60	29	17	11
Derive <35% food energy from total fat	50	14	40	35
Obesity	<7	10		
Men drinking >21 units alcohol/week	17	34		
Women drinking >14 units alcohol/week	6	11		

consumption of 35% compared with present day levels of 40%. Present evidence is that intakes of other fatty acids should not increase to compensate for the reduction in saturated fatty acids so that total fat has to decrease.

Currently, 10% of the adult British population is obese, a proportion which has increased from 7% in 1980.[8 9] For its third target, the green paper proposes a reversal of this trend so that the proportion of obese adults should again return to 7% by 2005. This is equivalent to about a 2 kg reduction in average weight, which could easily be achieved by a few extra minutes a day spent walking. The proposed reduction in total fat consumption alone would be more than sufficient to provide the daily 16 kJ energy deficit necessary to achieve the targeted weight reduction within 10 years as low fat diets do not favour fat storage and the energy cost of storage is higher.[10]

The fourth goal is for a reduction in alcohol consumption towards the recommended safe levels of 14 units a week for women and 21 units for men. Alcohol may account for hypertension in 10-15% of patients,[3] and alcoholic drinks have been graded by the WHO International Agency for Research on Cancer as a group 1 carcinogen in cancer of the oral cavity, pharynx, larynx, oesophagus and liver.[11]

Overall, the dietary goals set out in the green paper are based on credible data, and they will be widely welcomed by all who have an interest in improving health. They are open to amendment in the light of recently published recommendations on starch, non-starch polysaccharides, salt, and sugars.[4] Adoption of these recommendations will assist in reaching other targets such as the control of diabetes and its complications, reduction in dental caries, and an increase in fruit and vegetable consumption. A healthy diet including fruits and vegetables is acknowledged to be important in reducing preventable deaths and ill health in pregnant women, infants, and children.[1]

No dietary goals have been set for prevention of cancer, with reliance instead placed on screening for breast and cervical cancer and stopping smoking to reduce mortality and ill health. The green paper acknowledges that diet is responsible for at least 10% of cancers, although attributable risk is presently put at 35%, with a maximum of 75%.[12] The recent Committeee on Medical Aspects of Food Policy report recommends a 50% increase in consumption of non-starch polysaccharides, which fits well with current recommendations, based on preliminary data, to increase fruit, vegetable, cereal, and fibre consumption. In case-control studies these foods all seem to reduce the risk of bowel, oesophageal, lung, and gastric cancer. The effects of fat, meat, and salt remain uncertain, but recommendations to reduce saturated and total fat may also help to reduce the risk of cancers.[13]

Meeting the targets

What are the consequences of these targets on the nation's choice of food? Table II sets out possible ways in which average diets could be altered to meet these goals and the dietary recommended values. To achieve the recommended values for non-starch polysaccharides, starch, and sugar vegetable consumption needs to be doubled and fruit, bread, and potato consumption needs to be increased by at least 50%. Towards reducing intake of saturated fatty acids by about 13 g a simple change from full fat to semi-skimmed milk and from full fat to low fat spreads will reduce fat consumption by 6 g. A change from average fat to lean meat might achieve a further 3 g reduction, and halving consumption of biscuits, cakes, puddings, chips, crisps, and chocolate (which currently supply 24% of the total intake of saturated fatty acids) would achieve the remaining 4 g. Consumption of soft drinks and table sugar would need to be halved to make the necessary 25 g reduction in non-milk extrinsic sugars. By definition, half the population will need to make more and half make less than these changes, with older age groups requiring greater changes because serum cholesterol concentrations, body weight, and saturated fat consumption are all greater in these groups than in 25-34 year olds.[8]

Changing eating habits

Are such changes achievable? Present evidence suggests that their adoption is unlikely to be achieved by dissemination of information from guidelines, booklets, and advice by health educators alone. There have been some recent changes in the British diet, such as increased sales of skimmed milk, low fat spreads, and wholemeal bread, yet intakes of fat as a percentage of total energy have apparently not decreased.[14] A system of nutritional surveillance of individual dietary intakes is now in place, and this will be invaluable in monitoring any progress after the adoption of these proposals.

The political acceptance of the need to change food habits in England does, however, mean that progress is possible in making sure these goals are met. Rationing of the food supply, or taxation of saturated fats and sucrose is hardly a political alternative, but there are

TABLE II — Possible change in average consumption of foods to achieve government targets for 2005 and dietary recommended values[4]

Food	Present intake[8] (g)	Possible future intake (g)	Contributions to required alterations in				Proportional change in intake
			Saturated fatty acids (g)	Non-milk extrinsic sugars (g)	Non-starch poly-saccharides (g)	Starch and other sugars (g)	
Wholemeal and other bread	43	110			2·2	50	2·5
White bread	65	85			0·3	10	1·3
Vegetables	135	270			3·0	11	2·0
Fruit	73	110			0·3	4	1·5
Potatoes	132	200			0·8	13	1·5
Biscuits, cakes, puddings	80	40	−2·4	−8			0·5
Whole to semi-skimmed milk	164	164	−2·0				1·0
Saturated to low fat spreads	10	10	−4·0				1·0
Meat to leaner meat	150	150	−3·0				1·0
Chips, crisps and change to lower fat products	62	31	−1·2				0·5
Chocolate	9	5	−0·7	−2			0·5
Sugar, preserves	23	12		−12			0·5
Beverages, soft drinks	100	50		−3			0·5
Total			−13	−25	6·5	88*	

*Includes allowance for the reduction in sources of non-milk extrinsic sugars.

less oppressive ways in which legislation could effect changes in food habits.

Firstly, the importance of nutrition must be re-established in the nation's mind, from schoolchildren onwards. The national palate needs re-educating, and healthy cooking and food choice must be taught. Low fat cookery needs special skills in, for example, the use of herbs and spices and low fat sauces and in vegetable cookery; a wide variety of fresh, different, healthy, and inexpensive foods have become available in recent years. Curriculums in schools and for caterers should devote more attention to this and less to traditional cookery methods, which usually require a lot of fat. Catering contracts to hospitals and possibly educational institutions could include legal requirements to provide food which meets the target levels, on a par with current regulations on food hygiene.

The consumer also needs to know what is in packaged food. Food labelling should become mandatory and include ready made and possibly restaurant meals. Supermarkets can assist consumers by displaying low fat foods in prominent areas and by possibly introducing designated "healthy shopping" areas. More dietitians need to be trained and available to assist food manufacturers, retailers, the media, and caterers in changing eating habits, and sufficient dietitians must be available to talk directly to patients and the public. Reliance on the dissemination of advice by other health professionals is unsatisfactory because their training in nutrition has been neglected. In one survey, 90% of medical students and doctors thought that their present education in nutrition was inadequate.[15]

Lastly, the possibility of curbing or opposing the massive amount of advertising for unhealthy food and drink must be considered. Regular television screening within the home goes a long way to overturning the hard work of all those presently participating in health education.

Future targets

And what of the future? There are enormous gaps in our knowledge of exactly how much and how diet contributes to the cause and prevention of many other diseases, such as cancer. These gaps exist because nutrition research has been neglected since its heyday in the 1920s and 1930s. Only about 3% of the Medical Research Council's budget is currently allocated to nutrition related research. It is to be hoped that a political decision to invest in improved health through

25

dietary measures will increase our knowledge of the effects of diet through adequate funding for medical aspects of nutrition.

1 Department of Health. *The health of the nation*. London, HMSO, 1991.
2 Department of Health and Human Science. *Surgeon General's report on nutrition and health*. Washington, DC: DHHS, 1988. (Publication 88-50210.)
3 World Health Organisation. Diet, nutrition and the prevention of chronic diseases. *WHO Tech Rep Ser* 1990. No 797.
4 Committee on Medical Aspects of Food Policy. *Dietary reference values for food energy and nutrients for the United Kingdom*. London: HMSO, 1991.
5 Shaper AG. *Coronary heart disease, risks and reasons*. London: Current Medical Literature, 1988.
6 Willett W. *Nutritional epidemiology*. New York: Oxford University Press, 1990.
7 Leaf A, Weber PC. Cardiovascular effects of n-3 fatty acids. *N Engl J Med* 1988;**318**:549-57.
8 Gregory J, Foster K, Tyler H, Wiseman M. *The dietary and nutritional survey of adults*. London: OPCS, 1990.
9 Knight I. *The heights and weights of adults in Great Britain*. London: HMSO, 1984.
10 Lean MEJ, James WPT. Metabolic effects of isoenergetic nutrient exchange over 24 hours in relation to obesity in women. *Int J Obes* 1988;**12**:15-27.
11 International Agency for Research on Cancer. *Monograph on evaluation of carcinogenic risks to humans*. Vol 44. *Alcohol drinking*. Lyons: IARC, 1988.
12 Doll R, Peto R. Quantitative estimates of avoidable risks of cancer in the US today. *J Natl Cancer Inst* 1981;**66**:1192-308.
13 Bingham S. *Diet and cancer briefing paper*. London: Health Education Authority, 1990.
14 Buss DH. Is the British diet improving? *Proc Nutr Soc* 1988;**47**:295-306.
15 Brett A, Godden DJ, Keenan R. Nutritional knowledge of medical staff and students. *Human Nutrition Applied Nutrition* 1986;**40A**:217-22.

Rehabilitation

D L McLELLAN

Rehabilitation is a very large subject for this format. The case that it should be a key area in the government's strategy may be summarised as follows:

- People with disabilities are numerous and their needs great
- The benefits of appropriate intervention are an improvement in the duration and quality of life
- Intervention also improves the contribution that people with disabilities can make to their community and reduces the needs of informal carers
- The government's criteria in *The Health of the Nation*[1] specifically justify including rehabilitation (box).

The recent surveys by the Office of Population Censuses and Surveys have shown that disability is common and has a profound effect on disposable income, employment, and quality of life.[4] The most common disabling conditions affect the musculoskeletal system and the special senses, but the greatest dependency results from neurological disorders, especially those that cause impaired cognitive function and behaviour in addition to physical disability. Although 10% of the general population have a disability of some kind, rehabilitation medicine services concentrate mainly on people with severe disabilities. These people include the 1000 or so in each health district between the ages of 16 and 65 who are unable to live at home for 24 hours or more without the physical help of another person—a group I shall subsequently refer to as people with appreciable dependency.[5] This group probably has the greatest risk of avoidable complications and deterioration such as deformities, accidental injury, intercurrent infection, pressure sores, and poor levels of

27

Government criteria including rehabilitation as a key area

- A major theme of the document is to find the right balance between "the three key areas: prevention, treatment and rehabilitation"
- Avoidable disability, illness, and premature death are themselves key targets
- Because rehabilitation is served by health related activities in many government departments it tends to be marginalised. The challenge of identifying objectives with solutions that require collaboration between departments is specifically accepted
- Objectives and targets can be set which will enable progress to be made
- Rehabilitation is specifically identified as an area with clear scope for improvement.[2] This is not only a matter of more resources but also of better targeting towards needs that are seen as important by the disabled person
- "Above all there is the need to maintain the quality of care and support for chronically sick people . . . and handicapped people . . . in the face of some significant demographic changes."[3]
- "There is a need for specific initiatives to address the health needs of particularly vulnerable groups . . . who need specific targeted help."
- Specific interventions that offer significant improvement in outcome are readily available

physical fitness. They are also prone to excess psychological stress, as are their informal carers and families. At the other end of the scale are people who have a considerable health related handicap despite successful medical or surgical treatment, the most notable example being people with epilepsy, whose difficulty in obtaining employment is out of all proportion to the disability experienced.[6]

Some of the interventions of rehabilitation medicine are self evidently effective, such as training wheelchair users in the prevention of pressure sores and the skilled use of communication aids for people who cannot talk. Despite the lack of resources allocated to research in rehabilitation there is increasing evidence of effectiveness in its whole range from the outcomes of coordinated programmes for people with spinal cord injuries[7] and the effects of neglect on disabled teenagers[8] to the impact of specific measures to improve communication and develop cognitive strategies that circumvent the effects of cognitive impairment.[9][10]

The case against rehabilitation being a key area

Neglect sets a precedent. Most medical graduates are profoundly ignorant of rehabilitation medicine and will readily identify priorities in other medical disciplines. Little research is funded by the government or by major charities in rehabilitation despite the difficulties of conducting research in this subject. It would be nice to think that this is because the problems of rehabilitation medicine have all been sorted out—but regrettably, it is simply evidence of marginalisation and neglect.

What should the targets be?

The first thing to be said is that many people with disabilities have their own targets.[11] Those that the Department of Health adopts should result from a process of discussion and negotiation in which people with disabilities are fully involved. I suggest that they should establish that the potential for personal rehabilitation has been realised, that an optimal level of function is maintained, and that the need for support of informal carers has been minimised.

To establish that the potential for personal rehabilitation has been realised, unrealised potential must be identified. Despite the impressive advances in techniques for doing this—for example, the Edinburgh rehabilitation index[12]—doubt will always exist in relation to individual people. Outcome measures therefore need to apply either to averaged values derived from the relevant population or to percentages of people within the population who reach the required outcome targets.

Locomotion and mobility, the capacity for self care, communication, and employment are key factors in target setting because of the impact they have on the quality of life and the demands they make on services.[3] For those incapable of open paid employment we need an indicator of whether their time is occupied in fulfilling activities. For carers outcome should particularly test their degree of stress and the restrictions imposed on their personal lives. We need easily identified targets that can be applied to as representative a proportion of the client group as possible, and we need to test the combined effects of all the principal contributors to the service. Defining outcomes for specific diseases or the effects of specific interventions is easier. The advantage of setting broadly based targets, however, is that careful attention will need to be paid to all the factors influencing the outcome of individual cases to be certain of reaching the target for the population as a whole. In this way the very process of measuring the outcome and planning how to meet the target will ensure that a reasonably comprehensive assessment is carried out and that hard thinking about the issues occurs in health districts.

This is a new and welcome approach to planning. As many of the outcomes are not currently measured with any accuracy, targets will need to be set in terms of percentage improvements on present performance. Current performance will therefore have to be measured to establish whether targets have been met. This information will subsequently allow absolute targets to be set.

I therefore suggest percentage reduction targets to be reached by 1996. By then absolute values would be known for all health districts so that during the following four years absolute targets could be set nationally.

To provoke discussion I have selected eight straightforward targets and seven that are more controversial. As rehabilitation medicine is concerned specifically with people aged 16 to 65 years, I have assumed that rehabilitation targets for children, elderly people, and people with psychiatric disability and mental handicap will be identified by the other authors in this series.

Non-controversial targets

● The annual incidence of pressure sores occurring in hospitals and residential institutions within each health district should fall to 50% of current values
● The prevalence of pressure sores in all health districts should fall to 50% of current values
● The incidence of limb fractures occurring as a result of falls due to impairment of mobility should decline to 75% of current values
● The prevalence of daytime incontinence from all causes that is sufficiently severe to necessitate a change of clothing more often than three times a month should fall to 75% of current values
● The numbers of people who because of difficulty in articulation or phonation are unable to communicate effectively other than with their

relatives should fall to 75% of current values. People who communicate satisfactorily by using a communication aid are excluded

• The incidence of significant contractures (restricting the range of movement at the elbow, knee, or ankle joints by 20° or more) developing during treatment for any cause in hospital should fall to 60% of current values in terms of both the number of limbs and the number of patients affected

• After traumatic brain injury the incidence of disturbances of behaviour requiring sedatives or major tranquillising drugs for more than 48 hours within six months after the injury should fall to 60% of current values

• The prevalence of carers of appreciably dependent people for whom sleep is interrupted on two or more occasions a night on three or more nights a week in order to help or supervise the disabled person should decline to 70% of current values.

Controversial targets

• The prevalence of obligative wheelchair users who because of their physical impairment are unable without the help of another person to leave and enter their home and to travel up to 1000 m outside their home should decline to 75% of current values

• The prevalence of people with appreciable visual impairment who because of their disability are unable without the help of another person to leave and enter their home and to travel up to 1000 m outside their home should decline to 75% of current values

• The rate of employment for people with disabilities, registered and unregistered, whose form UBI671 indicates that they have a disability or health problem that restricts the nature or amount of work they can do should fall from $2 \cdot 8 \times$ the rate for non-disabled people to $2 \cdot 0 \times$ the rate for non-disabled people in all employment department regions

• The incidence of clinical depression occurring during the first year of recovery from stroke or spinal cord injury should decline to 75% of current values

• The number of people who because of their physical disability are unable unless physically assisted by another person to visit their dentist or their general practitioner in his or her surgery should fall to zero

• The prevalence of clinical anxiety or depression in the main informal carers of appreciably dependent people should fall to 75% of current values

• The prevalence of clinical anxiety or depression in the main

31

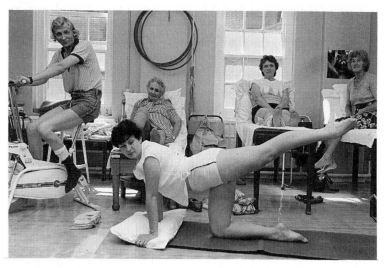

Though rehabilitation for people with acute disabilities is good, services for those with chronic illness or disability are scarce

informal carers of people who have had a severe or very severe head injury within the previous five years should fall to 75% of current values.

What should be the strategy for reaching the targets?

To achieve these targets a rehabilitation task force should be set up in each district with an experienced manager supported by a small group that includes representatives of disabled people and senior professional staff from health, social, and local authority services. Hospitals would be required to identify people and audit the objectives in the following categories:

● People who habitually use crutches, walking frames, or wheelchairs for mobility who have been admitted with a stroke, head injury, pressure sores, spinal cord injury, and limb fractures

● Patients who develop the sentinel events of pressure sores or contractures in hospital

● People recovering from severe or very severe head injury who either develop contractures or require psychotropic drugs. (Though essential for management in some cases, drugs are frequently an ineffective substitute for more humane methods of behavioural management.)

Community services would be required to identify and monitor annually six groups of people:

- Those needing to use a wheelchair for all journeys outside their home
- Those recovering from a moderate or severe head injury within the previous five years
- Those who are appreciably dependent
- Those with severe impairment of vision
- Those with dysarthria severe enough to prevent communication except with family members
- The main informal carers of appreciably dependent people.

This would ensure the effective monitoring and selected audit of the objectives for some of the most vulnerable categories of people with disabilities, including most of those who have been the subject of recent public concern — namely, disabled school leavers, people with multiple disabilities including the effects of head injury, and carers. The very process of monitoring and feedback is likely to improve outcome.[13] I have no space to detail the precise interventions (most of which are self evident) that could help meet these targets. Success on the initial targets could be achieved by improvement in only some components of the service, but full success on the subsequent targets would require effective collaboration and combined action between rehabilitation medicine services in hospital and the community services, social services, housing, transport, and employment departments in each district. By 1996 enough information should be available to enable absolute targets to be set for each component of the overall rehabilitation service (allowing comparison between different districts) for the period from 1996 to the year 2000.

What will be the problems in achieving these targets?

One problem in achieving these targets is that the targets themselves will be seen as arbitrary and excluding a lot of people with urgent needs. The present period of discussion is to help us define priorities. Once the targets are agreed our main problems will be obtaining informed commitment from NHS management and in funding the task groups needed to monitor and implement them. In most districts the skill needed is already available but is either too thinly spread or working too much in isolation to be effective.

In addition these targets are not scientifically or conceptually complex. They call for shrewdness and imagination on the part of directors of community health medicine, precision in the operation of rehabilitation sevices, and the ability of all concerned to work across professional and service boundaries in the interests of disabled people. Sniping between professions and, of course, lack of unity between the medical profession and disabled people about the importance of the final list of objectives are pitfalls we should be able to avoid. Can we really afford not to succeed?

1 Secretary of State for Health. *The health of the nation*. London: HMSO, 1991. (Cm 1523.)
2 Edwards FC, Warren MD. *Health services for adults with physical disabilities. A survey of district health authorities, 1988/89*. London: Royal College of Physicians, 1990.
3 Robine JM, Ritchie K. Healthy life expectancy: evaluation of global indicator of change in population health. *BMJ* 1991;**302**:457-60.
4 Office of Population Censuses and Surveys. *Survey of disability in Great Britain*. Vols 1-6. London: HMSO, 1988, 1989.
5 Cantrell EG, Dawson J, Glastonbury G. *Prisoners of handicap*. London: RADAR, 1985.
6 McLellan DL. Epilepsy and employment. *J Soc Occup Med* 1987;**37**:94-9.
7 Alexander JL, Willens EP, Halstead LS, Spencer WA. The relationship of functional assessment to evaluation of the quality of outcome in the rehabilitation process. In: Alperovitch A, de Dombal ST, Gremy S, eds. *Evaluation of efficacy of medical action*. Amsterdam: North Holland Publishing, 1979:287-307.
8 Thomas AP, Bax M, Smyth DP. *The health and social needs of young adults with physical disabilities*. London: MacKeith Press, 1989. (Clinics in Developmental Medicine No 106.)
9 Wilson BA. Future directions in the rehabilitation of brain injured people. In: Christensen A-L, Uzzell BP, eds. *Neuropsychological rehabilitation*. Amsterdam; Kluwer, 1988:69-86.
10 Godfrey HPD, Knight RG. Memory training and behavioural rehabilitation of a severely head-injured adult. *Arch Phys Med Rehabil* 1988;**69**:458-60.
11 Beardshaw V. *Last on the list. Community services for people with physical disabilities*. London: King's Fund, 1988.
12 Cornes P, Roy CW. Vocational rehabilitation index assessment of rehabilitation medicine service patients. *Int Disabil Stud* 1991;**13**:5-9.
13 Carpenter GI, Demopoulos GR. Screening the elderly in the community: controlled trial of dependency surveillance using a questionnaire administered by volunteers. *BMJ* 1990;**300**: 1253-6.

Challenge of aging

J GRIMLEY EVANS

Our idea of what constitutes effectiveness and efficiency in the health and social services depends on whether we are customers or purveyors. In an obsession with cost accounting and the ethically questionable issue of how many quality adjusted life years (QALYs) can be bought for each taxpayer's pound,[1] the government has been offering an exclusively purveyor's agenda for assessing health and community care. It is therefore refreshing to find that *The Health of the Nation*[2] is mostly concerned with customer interests—health rather than health expenditure and health outcomes rather than service processes.

Curiously, however, given the realities of health care in our aging population, older people are conspicuously absent from most of its pages. Premature death is taken to be death before the age of 65, a definition recalling times when individuals were valued only as exploitable labour. This now seems anachronistic, if only because expectation of life at birth is 73 years for men and 78 for women.[2] It may also be less than astute politically given that people aged over 65 comprise a fifth of the electorate and sooner or later will start voting with their heads.

More promisingly for older people, the document proposes the identification of key areas that can be defined in terms of avoidable ill health , and, even more importantly, ill health is to include disability. Rehabilitation services for people with a physical disability are offered as a possible key area. This too is promising provided that citizens aged over 65 are to count as people. Unhappily the document considers rehabilitation in the context of a publication from the Royal College of Physicians that did not include geriatric rehabilitation in its considerations. This could hardly be less timely. Experience from the

35

US warns that under the contractual prepayment system of the reformed NHS, one way that managers will seek to trim hospital costs will be by withdrawing rehabilitation from older patients.[3] The brief paragraph dealing specifically with older people is ambiguous and possibly misconceived (box). Although the importance of a healthier old age is recognised, the document offers no programme for ensuring good health in elderly people and age associated disability is not suggested as a key area. (Age associated is a descriptive term with no implication that the disability is caused by intrinsic aging[4] or is an inevitable accompaniment of age).

Storing up ill health

Two messages seem to emerge from all this: the first, for the general public, is that the government's concern for the human sufferings caused by ill health in old age is primarily the associated nuisance created in a demand for services; the second, for the professions, is that preventive medicine is viewed simply as postponement of disease to an age when further avoidance becomes impossible and the cumulated backlog falls finally and, by implication, inevitably. It would be charitable to assume that these are false messages produced by maladroit drafting, but the second message offers a coherent epidemiological model that can be judged on its merits.

The incidence of most diseases increases with age, and in the case of

---

Green paper strategy for elderly people

Between 1981 and 1989 the number of people aged 75-84 has risen by 16%, and those 85 and over by 39%. . . . Much of what this document says about prevention of heart disease, stroke and cancers is especially relevant to this growing number of elderly people. This is where the burden of avoidable ill-health finally falls. The government recognises, moreover, that success in reducing premature mortality will increase the number of elderly people and so, unless a healthier old age accompanies greater longevity, lead to a greater demand for services. That is why the emphasis must be as much on quality of life as on quantity of life.

some important preventable diseases such as cancers and stroke incidence shows a power-law relation to age[5 6]; with others such as proximal femoral fracture the relation is exponential. In general when incidence differs because of some extrinsic cause, and cohort effects are corrected for, the slope of the incidence curve remains the same but its intercept changes. The overall incidence of proximal femoral fracture measured in Oxford in 1966 and in Newcastle upon Tyne in 1975-6 differed by a factor of two but the exponential curves in the two studies were parallel.[7] There was no increased steepness in the Oxford data to suggest that fractures were being "stored up" into later ages. Mortality from stroke has been falling at similar proportional rates in both middle aged and older people.[8] The evidence therefore suggests that reducing extrinsic causes of disease will prevent some people from getting a disease rather than merely postponing the age at which they get it.

Disease may not be avoided, however, if preventive measures are not continued into later life. Healthy lifestyles are associated with increased longevity at the age of 70 as at younger ages,[9] though we do not yet know that the association is causal. There is increasing evidence of the predictive power of risk factors for vascular disease in old age.[10 11] The research necessary to assess the efficacy of risk factor modulation in later life must be carried out. But in the real world of medicine our ethical duty is to "manfully act upon the greater probability,"[12] and many gerontologists will feel that the burden of proof lies with those who want to treat elderly people differently from middle aged people in regard to prevention of disease. Certainly, such an attitude will be a more potent encouragement to government funded research than would the cheaper null hypothesis.

Health of elderly people as a key area

The Health of the Nation sets out clearly and reasonably what should be the criteria for identifying a key area; briefly it should be a major cause of concern and there should be scope for improvement for which targets can be set. Nearly 60% of disabled people in Britain are aged 65 and over,[13] and age associated disability is by any standard a major cause for concern. Differences in the prevalence of disability among definable social groups, in this country and elsewhere, together with evidence of the variation in incidence of disabling diseases such as stroke and proximal femoral fracture are clear

37

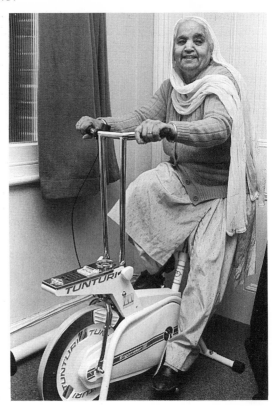

Unless
increased longevity
is accompanied by
good health demands
on services will grow

indicators that improvements could be realistically looked and planned for.

The government's proposed approach to disability includes a focus on specific disabilities and impairments such as incontinence and pressure sores. For older people we now have a more global approach to measuring disability of all forms that could be used for target setting. This is the concept of active life expectancy,[14] in which life expectancy at any age is divided into average years left before death and average years left before disability intervenes. With routine data measures of active life expectancy often have to be approximated by measures of independent life expectancy—that is, years until the first use of informal or statutory help from others. Such measures are susceptible to bias from the availability of the services identified as defining dependency. Active life expectancy defined in terms of disability could be monitored in representative population groups by standardised and repeated surveys of abilities to perform specified tasks of daily living. A project of the Central Health Monitoring Unit in cooperation with the Office of Populations Censuses and Surveys is to be welcomed as providing a pilot for studies of this kind. Furthermore, it is not too fanciful to conceive of a time when the improved surveillance of elderly people recently introduced in primary care, together with computerised databases in primary care, could be used to monitor independent life expectancy in later life on a nationwide basis. This possibility is foreseen by the health services research committee of the Medical Research Council in expressing interest in the development of an effective system for use in the mandatory primary care surveillance of older people.

Active life expectancy could be increased by prevention or intervention, or both. A modest target would be that active life expectancy at age 65 should increase in its proportion of total life expectancy and by a specified annual percentage. A health authority could decide on the basis of local information how best to distribute its efforts between different possible activities in order to achieve this. For example, one authority might aim at reducing strokes by a programme of blood pressure control in later life; another might decide to improve its hip replacement programme.

Separatist or integrationist strategy?

The case for recognising age associated disability as one of the government's key areas seems to be at least as cogent as that for some other topics suggested. Indeed, some will see its omission as positively anomalous. Assuming that the government has not cynically ignored a politically inactive section of the population, or failed to do its homework, what are the counterarguments?

One could invoke the longstanding dilemma of whether older people should be identified as a special group or merely as people who may have problems that the health and social services should be able to deal with whatever the age of the patient. This difference in philosophy has distinguished the "separatist" and the "integrationist" wings of geriatric medicine for nearly two decades, but the integrationists have never suggested that the needs of older people could be ignored. The essence of the integrationist philosophy has always been that services should be deployed according to need rather than age and must be as suitable for elderly people as for young. If the government were proposing an integrationist strategy, it should have made clear that elderly people were included in its focus on disability, rehabilitation, and preventable death. In fact elderly people have been implicitly excluded.

Whatever the reasons *The Health of the Nation* is surprisingly inadequate in its response to the challenge of our aging population. There is likely to be a more or less respectful clamour for the health problems of older people to be designated, in one form or other, as a key area in what is an important and exciting initiative. So debased has the coinage of public debate become that many will suspect that *The Health of the Nation* is merely a political document saying what the government thinks the public might like to hear in the run up to a general election. The government's willingness to enlarge its list of key areas to include age associated disability would be a significant demonstration of its genuineness in producing a consultative document.

1 Harris J. QALYfying the value of life. *J Med Ethics* 1987;**13**:117-23.
2 Secretary of State for Health. *The health of the nation.* London: HMSO, 1991. (Cm 1523.)
3 Fitzgerald JF, Moore PS, Dittus RS. The care of elderly patients with hip fracture. Changes since implementation of the prospective payment system. *N Engl J Med* 1988;**319**:1392-7.
4 Fairweather DS, Grimley Evans J. Ageing. In: Cohen RD, Lewis B, Alberti KGMM, Denman AM, eds. *The metabolic and molecular basis of acquired disease.* Vol 1. London: Baillière Tindall, 1991:213-36.
5 Doll R. The age distribution of cancer: implications for models of carcinogenesis. *Journal of the Royal Statistical Society* 1971;**134**[A]:133-55.
6 Grimley Evans J, Caird FI. Epidemiology of neurological disorders in old age. In: Caird FI, ed. *Neurological disorders in the elderly.* Bristol: Wright, 1982: 1-16.
7 Rees JL. Secular changes in the incidence of proximal femoral fracture in Oxfordshire: a preliminary report. *Community Medicine* 1982;**4**:100-3.
8 Grimley Evans J. The decline of stroke. In: Rose FC, ed. *Stroke: epidemiological, therapeutic and socio-economic aspects.* London: Royal Society of Medicine, 1986:33-8.
9 Branch LG, Jette AM. Personal health practices and mortality among the elderly. *Am J Public Health* 1984;**74**:1126-9.
10 Khaw K-T. Serum lipids in later life. *Age Ageing* 1990;**19**:277-90.
11 Beaglehole R. Coronary heart disease and elderly people. *BMJ* 1991;**303**: 69-70.
12 Acland H. *Memoir of the cholera at Oxford in the year 1854.* Oxford, 1854.
13 Office of Population Censuses and Surveys. *Survey of disability in Great Britain.* London: HMSO, 1988.
14 Katz S, Branch LG, Branson MH, Papsidero JA, Beck JC, Greer DS. Active life expectancy. *N Engl J Med* 1983;**309**:1218-24.

Mental health

GRAHAM THORNICROFT,
GERALDINE STRATHDEE

The green paper *The Health of the Nation*[1] presents an opportunity to forge a practical and ambitious strategy for the development of English mental health services into the twenty first century. Its structure encourages clarity of purpose, specificity of interventions, and accuracy in measuring outcomes of treatment, and this we applaud. We do not, however, agree that "it is unrealistic to set health outcome targets for these services." Indeed, it is through setting targets that we may now promote the central place of mental health in a healthy nation.

Historically mental health issues have been marginalised within medical practice. Two recent examples illustrate this point. The World Health Organisation's programme Health for All by the year 2000 includes only one mental health goal within the 38 areas—to reduce suicide rates.[2] Similarly, only 13 of 133 English districts recently surveyed mentioned mental health matters in their 1989 public health reports.[2] This neglect is unwarranted. Mental health planners and practitioners already have tools to measure the success of much of their work.[4][5] The onus should be on psychiatrists at the local level to pursue active collaboration with public health doctors to identify local needs and to plan services.

In our view, however, mental health targets should extend beyond mental illness services, and should include the domains of prevention, promotion, and the psychosocial aspects of general health care.[6] These last three domains have been underemphasised in the NHS, and contributions are needed from colleagues across a wide spectrum of interests to join debate on these aspects of mental health policy. In this chapter we shall focus on the psychiatric treatment and care of

41

adults, accepting that parallel initiatives are needed in related fields, including the mental health of children, families, and elderly people.

Why should mental health be a key area?

The green paper requires key areas to be justified in terms of the burdens of mortality, morbidity, and cost. Although death is not often seen as an adverse outcome of mental illness, the all cause mortality for schizophrenia, for example, is estimated to be over twice that of the general population,[7] principally attributable to suicide, accidents, and cardiovascular disorders. The extent of psychiatric illness in the population is sobering.[8 9] Surveys in primary care have shown that at least 26% of the population consult their family doctor each year with a mental health problem.[10] In addition, there is considerable illness among patients' relatives and care givers, who often develop psychiatric symptoms from their burden of care.[11]

The costs of mental ill health are also staggering: these problems account for 14% of days lost to work, 20% of total NHS expenditure, 23% of inpatient costs, and 25% of pharmaceutical charges.[1] The total annual costs of mental illness are estimated at £4·6-£5·6 billion,[12 13] less than a third of which is for direct services. Mental illness, therefore, amply fulfils the three criteria necessary to qualify as a key area.

What should mental health targets be?

We support the overall objective of the green paper "to reduce the level of disability caused by mental illness by improving significantly the treatment and care of mentally disordered people," but we want services that are local and accessible, comprehensive, flexible, culturally and ethnically appropriate, accountable, equitably distributed, and based on need and that offer continuity of treatment and care.[14 15]

The government's single target is "To realign the resources currently spent on specialist psychiatric services into district based services, thereby allowing many of the remaining 90 psychiatric hospitals . . . to be closed."[1] We believe that this target needs amplifying and propose that mental health targets be set at five levels of intervention; responsibilities should be defined at national, regional, district health authority or family health services authority, provider, and patient levels. Tables I-V detail our proposed targets for each

TABLE I—National targets and indicators for mental health

Target	Indicators
Develop measures of progress toward national mental health objectives	1 Develop standard national descriptions of mental health service components by 1 January 1993 2 Publish an annual national mental health report from 1 January 1993 including (a) the number and rank order of day, residential, inpatient, day patient, outpatient, and home care facilities in each district and (b) the number of patients detained under the Mental Health Act
Continue hospital rundown programme	1 45 Of the hospitals now with over 400 beds to close by 2000 2 No psychiatric hospital to have over 400 beds by 1995 and none over 250 beds by 2000. 3 Specific transitional funding arrangements to be provided by Department of Health to regions 4 The proportion of mental health expenditure on local facilities to increase by 40% by 1995 and by 60% by 2000
Reduce preventable deaths	1 Reduce the number of former patients committing suicide by 10% by 2000. 2 Reduce standardised mortality ratio among schizophrenic patients by 10% by 2000 3 Provide health education on smoking to 50% of psychiatric patients by 1995 and to 90% by 2000 4 Increase the proportion of psychiatric units operating no smoking policies to 50% by 1995 and 90% by 2000
Structural requirements	1 Establish long term and serious mental illness as the national priority group for mental illness services 2 Establish ringfenced health and social services budgets by 1 April 1993 3 Establish clear mental health definitions—for example, for long term and serious mental illness 4 Convene a national mental health commission by 1 January 1993 to oversee annual mental health report 5 Establish a national mental health resources centre by 1 October 1993

TABLE II—Regional targets and indicators for mental health

Target	Indicators
Develop measures of progress toward regional mental health objectives	1 Annual regional mental health report with common core information 2 Increase proportion of community to hospital expenditure by 40% by 1995
Continue hospital rundown programme	1 45 Of the hospitals now with over 400 beds to close by 2000 2 No pysychiatric hospital to have over 400 beds by 1995 and none over 250 beds by 2000 3 The proportion of mental health expenditure on local facilities to increase by 40% by 1995 and by 60% by 2000
Structural requirements	1 Ringfenced regional mental health budgets 2 Establish local manpower requirements

TABLE III—Mental health targets and indicators for district health authorities and family health services authorities

Target		Indicators
Develop measures of progress toward district mental health objectives	1	Annual district public health report by 1 October 1992 with common core information
Develop locally based services	1	Over 90% of catchment area patients treated in district health authority by 1995, over 95% by 2000
	2	Increase proportion of community expenditure by 40% by 1995 and by 60% by 2000
	3	Set minimum requirements for provision of day care places by 1 October 1992
	4	Set minimum requirements for sheltered residential places by 1 October 1992 (for example, 100 places/100 000 population as in Cambridge)
	5	Increase proportion of community to hospital staff by 40% by 1995 and 60% by 2000
	6	Reduce number of inpatients with psychosis who have been in hospital for over 6 months and 1 year by 20% by 1995 and 40% by 2000
	7	Set target proportion of former patients with psychosis in contact with services and on local case register at 75% by 1995.
	8	Set target proportion of mentally abnormal offenders who are treated in district services by 1995. Set maximum waiting times for mentally abnormal offenders in special hospitals and at regional secure units to return to district facilities
	9	Increase number of community mental health teams in each district
	10	Increase number of community psychiatric nurses who have received training in working with long term patients
	11	Reduce number of days by which 50%, 75%, and 90% of patients had been discharged
Structural requirements	1	Ringfenced budgets
	2	Establish joint local mental health strategic plans
	3	Ensure user representation at local planning level by 1 January 1992
	4	Complete needs assessments on over 90% of patients in target groups (for example, homeless mentally ill) by 1 April 1993
Develop liaison between primary and secondary care levels	1	Increase proportion of psychiatrists working in primary care settings by 20% by 1995
	2	Continuing training for over 20% of general practitioners in the treatment of serious mental illnesses by 1 October 1993

level. The targets and their indicators are intended to stimulate debate between health and social agencies, service users, and the voluntary sector so that ambitious and detailed targets for mental health can be incorporated into the white paper.

The targets cover structure, process, and outcome. In terms of

TABLE IV—Mental health targets and indicators for providers

Target	Indicators
Structural requirements	1 Relevant discharge and care programme plans completed for 90% of patients with psychosis and organic mental disorder by 1995
	2 Establish local information systems of vulnerable patients by 1 January 1993
Service characteristics	1 Managed multidisciplinary community care and hospital teams in each unit by 1 April 1993
	2 Clear written local service objectives with rank of priorities by each unit by 1 April 1992
	3 Increase proportion of face to face interagency contact by 10% by 1 January 1993
	4 Decrease proportion of patients with joint care plans who have not contacted service in past 6 months
	5 Increase proportion of long term patients in sheltered work or day care facilities
	6 Increase the proportion of patients receiving depot antipsychotic drugs who have a care programme with regular multidisciplinary reviews
	7 Less than 5% of acute beds occupied by patients staying over 60 days
	8 Less than 10% of discharge patients readmitted within 6 months

TABLE V—Mental health targets and indicators for patients

Target	Indicators
Measure clinical disability outcomes	1 Self rated symptom scales
	2 Interviewer administered symptoms scales
Measure social disability outcomes	1 Employment
	2 Social roles
	3 Social behaviour
Measure user assessments of services	1 Satisfaction with care
	2 Knowledge about services
	3 Relatives burden rating
	4 Quality of life measure

structure of service a consensus has emerged over the past decade on the characteristics that locally based services should assume.[16][17] Regions and districts should first make an inventory of the range, character, and size of local facilities and then draw up a timescale during which services should be reoriented towards specific targets. The evidence suggests that the worst of service provision is very poor. Most districts, for example, have no mental health respite care facilities.[18]

Process variables, although underemphasised in the green paper, may be crucial in tracking the function of services. Evidence from mental health centres, for example, suggests that policy targets will not be met unless the process of care is strictly monitored.[19] But perhaps the single most important change in process variables is to increase the proportion of the £1·5 billion NHS mental health budget that is spent on local mental health services. At present over half is spent on the 40 000 psychiatric patients remaining in hospital. If we conservatively estimate that about 180 000 (0·5%) of the 36 million adult population of England[20] suffer from severe forms of mental illness[21 22] then less than half the total expenditure reaches the 78% of severely disabled patients who live in the community.

Validated outcome variables are available for only some of the domains that require measurement (see table V), and investment is urgently needed in the construction and testing of further measures.[23 24] This task may fall within the remit of the new research and development division of the Department of Health and will allow brief and standardised measures to be disseminated to the local level. Methods have been established for measuring severity of symptoms, social behaviour, cognitive function, social role performance, needs assessment, and social networks. Further development is needed for measures of user knowledge and satisfaction and carer burden and for brief cost effectiveness rating scales.

What should the strategy be?

Nationally two prime structural issues must be addressed. Firstly, there is a lack of leadership, with no identified organisation taking responsibility for policy development and implementation. Instead policy is decided by a plurality of organisations with uncoordinated inputs including the Audit Commission, the Mental Health Act Commission, the Department of Health, the Royal College of Psychiatrists, and the Health Advisory Service.

Secondly, within government there is no formal mechanism for interdepartmental coordination of mental health policy. It has long been clear that social factors, which cut across usual departmental boundaries, have a key role in psychiatric morbidity.[25-27] Unemployment, for example, often produces an unacceptable level of anxiety, depression, self harm, and suicide.[28] The green paper officially recognises these health variations and proposes a pragmatic strategy that would formally integrate health and social policy. Such a ministerial grouping would necessarily include the Departments of Health, Social Security, and the Environment. An alternative strategy would be to set up a national mental health commission.

In either case the priorities would be to develop clear policies on provision of mental health service, to review the functions of the diverse organisations, to recommend how the organisations could be focused and coordinated more effectively, and to agree national standard definitions — for example, of serious mental illness, new long term patients, and types of residential care. A further priority should be to establish a national mental health resource centre to plan and implement community services and produce sophisticated and effective protocols to guide service developments, along the lines of the recent Social Services Inspectorate report on children and adolescent homes.[29]

There is a strong case for having regional task forces to support providers in auditing current practice and in preparing checklists against which local services can be appraised. The task forces could help local services look more systematically at process and outcome, set targets, and advise on management and service structures. Progress should be recorded according to a standard format in each annual regional public health report.

Another area of concern is the lack of provision for transitional service developments at each level of ringfenced, time limited funding. Provision needs to be made according to clearly formulated and rational guidelines. An example of poor practice is the recent introduction of the mental illness grant to social services departments; the lack of clarity and the inadequate time allowed for planning has led, in many instances, to cosmetic rather than radical innovations with little indication of outcomes.[30]

At district level one of the most fundamental barriers to rational planning and evaluation has been the lack of even basic infrastructures for obtaining information.[31][32] Strategic guidance from both regional and national levels has been minimal, and while local ownership of such systems is crucial to their success, the provision of expert consultants could expedite the development of systems more relevant to planning than the current performance indicators.

Locally purchasers may increasingly wish to use service specifications to insist on agreed priority groups of patients; measures of structure, process, and outcome; annual district public health reports including mental illness indicators in a standard format that allows direct comparisons across units; and providers actively pursuing close liaison between primary and secondary care services.[33]

These proposals go far beyond the single target set for mental health services in the green paper. They require a commitment at each level to accord mental health and mental illness services a priority never previously enjoyed. They raise the possibility that the Cinderella services may not necessarily return to dreary rags after the glitter of the green paper ball.

1 Secretary of State for Health. *The Health of the Nation*. London: HMSO, 1991.
2 World Health Organisation. *Global strategy for health for all by the year 2000*. Geneva: WHO, 1981.
3 Farrow S. Introduction to annual reports of public health. In: Jenkins R, Griffiths S, eds. *Indicators for mental health in the population*. London: HMSO, 1991: 1-5.
4 Thompson C. *The instruments of psychiatric reasearch*. Chichester: Wiley, 1989.
5 Wetzler S. *Measuring mental illness*. Washington, DC: American Psychiatric Press, 1989.
6 Sartorius N. Preface. In: Goldberg D, Tantam D, eds. *The public health impact of mental disorder*. Toronto: Hofgrefe and Huber, 1990: vii-xii.
7 Allebeck P. Schizophrenia: a life-shortening disease. *Schizophr Bull* 1989;**15**: 81-9.
8 Bebbington P, Hurry J, Tennant C, Sturt E, Wing J. Epidemiology of mental disorders in Camberwell. *Psychol Med* 1981;**11**:561-79.
9 Mann A. Public health and psychiatric morbidity. In: Jenkins R, Griffiths S, eds. *Indicators for mental health in the population*. London: HMSO, 1991: 6-17.
10 Goldberg D. Filter to care—a model. In: Jenkins R, Griffiths S, eds. *Indicators for mental health in the population*. London: HMSO, 1991: 30-7.
11 MacCarthy B, Lesage A, Brewin C, Brugha T, Wing J. Needs for care among the relatives of long term users of day care. *Psychol Med* 1989;**19**:725-36.
12 Croft-Jeffreys C, Wilkinson G. Estimated costs of neurotic disorder in the UK general practice, 1985. *Psychol Med* 1989;**19**:549-58.
13 Davies L, Drummond M. The economic burden of schizophrenia. *Br J Psychiatry* 1990;**154**: 522-5.
14 National Institutes of Mental Health. *Towards a model for a comprehensive community-based mental health system*. Washington, DC: NIMH, 1987.
15 MIND. *Common concern*. London: MIND Publications, 1983.
16 Murphy E. Community mental health services: a vision for the future. *BMJ* 1991;**302**:1064-5.
17 Leff J. Planning a community psychiatric service: from theory to practice. In: Wilkinson G, Freeman H, eds. *The provision of mental health services in Britain: the way ahead*. London: Gaskell, 1986: 49-60.
18 Thornicroft G. Are England's psychiatric services for schizophrenia improving? *Hosp Community Psychiatry* 1990;**41**:1073-5.
19 Patmore C, Weaver T. Rafts on an open sea. *Health Service Journal* 1990 October 11:1510-2.
20 Office of Population Censuses and Surveys. *Census 1981*. London: HMSO, 1983.
21 Goldman H. Defining and counting the chronically mentally ill. *Hosp Community Psychiatry* 1981;**32**:21-7.
22 Schinnar A, Rothbard A, Kanter R, Soo Jung Y. An empirical literature review of definitions of severe and persistent mental illness. *Am J Psychiatry* 1990;**147**:1602-8.
23 Jenkins R. Towards a system of outcome indicators for mental health care. *Br J Psychiatry* 1990;**157**:500-14.
24 Glover G, Farmer R, Preston D. Indicators of mental hospital bed use. *Health Trends* 1990;**22**:111-5.
25 Bruce M, Takeuchi D, Leaf P. Poverty and psychiatric status. *Arch Gen Psychiatry* 1991;**48**:470-4.
26 Thornicroft G. Social deprivation and rates of treated mental disorder: developing statistical models to predict psychiatric service utilisation. *Br J Psychiatry* 1991;**158**:475-84.
27 Hirsch S. *Psychiatric bed and resources: factors influencing bed use and service planning*. London: Gaskell, Royal College of Psychiatrists, 1988.
28 Warr P. *Unemployment, work and mental health*. Oxford: Oxford University Press, 1987.
29 Social Services Inspectorate. *Bridge over troubled waters*. London: Social Services Inspectorate, 1990.

30 Groves T. The mental illness grant. *BMJ* 1991;**302**:1416-7.
31 Wing J, ed. *Health services planning and research. Contributions from psychiatric case registers.* London: Gaskell, 1989.
32 World Health Organisation. *Implications for the field of mental health of the European targets for attaining health for all.* Copenhagen: WHO, 1991.
33 Strathdee G. The delivery of psychiatric care. *J R Soc Med* 1990;**83**:222-5.

Health of pregnant women

MARION H HALL

Reproduction is highly important for human well-being. Decisions about whether, when, and how to have children are of the utmost importance to individuals and inextricably entwined with the closest human relationships. Society does, however, have a legitimate interest in the birth of an appropriate number of children and in those children being as healthy as possible, including those with impairments. The health of pregnant women is thus an obvious aspect for consideration as a key area in a health strategy. The case for and against its selection will be discussed in respect of maternal, fetal, and neonatal mortality and morbidity and in the light of the potential for and feasibility of prevention.

Case for targets

Maternal mortality

The death of any pregnant woman or recently delivered mother is shocking to all concerned. Around 75 British women still die every year from pregnancy related causes, and the regional variation in the rate of pregnancy related death per 100 000 births varied from 5·8 to 10·6 among regions in the years 1976-87.[1] The regional variation may be partly due to maternal characteristics, but the report concludes that substandard care was provided in most cases, and at least some of these deaths may have been avoidable.

Maternal morbidity

Little or no routine data are collected on morbidity, though it may be assumed to be greater after caesarean section or instrumental delivery, and intervention rates are enormously variable. The extent of distress associated with perinatal death and miscarriage is now acknowledged. Taking a broad definition of health it could also be argued that unwanted pregnancy, resulting in termination, is a manifestation of ill health, and this now occurs in about one in five or six conceptions.

Fetal and neonatal mortality

Estimates in prospective studies of the likelihood of fetal death from conception to term vary from 13% to 24%,[2] and perinatal death, at 5-10 babies per 1000 births, is much commoner than death in the rest of childhood and early adult life. There are again considerable regional variations, more than could be explained by chance,[3] but the question of what proportion of deaths is avoidable is open.

Possible aims in the government's health strategy

The scope for safeguarding and improving the health of mothers (before, during, and after pregnancy) and of babies includes:

- Adoption of a healthy lifestyle—in particular good nutrition and avoidance of both smoking and more than minimal alcohol consumption during pregnancy
- Effective family planning services for those men and women who wish for this
- Protection against infectious diseases (for example, rubella)
- High quality maternity care services (tailored where appropriate to the needs of particularly vulnerable groups such as unsupported mothers and certain ethnic minorities)
- Improving management of obstetric emergencies by having available in every maternity unit a consultant obstetrician and anaesthetist whose main priorities are to oversee the labour ward
- Good infant nutrition
- Improving general socioeconomic and environmental circumstances, in particular quality of housing
- Health education and promotion (about all of the above)

Target: By 1993 all regional health authorities (and in turn district health authorities and family health services authorities) should have established targets for reducing stillbirths and infant deaths (possibly with separate targets for different causes).

51

Fetal morbidity

This is an appropriate aspect on which to focus services as it may result in a wide range of mental or physical impairments. The incidence of cerebral palsy, one of the most serious sequelae, has not fallen with perinatal death rates. The condition is thought to be due only rarely to birth asphyxia and possibly to early pregnancy influences, but it is strongly associated with birthweight.[4] The aetiology of some congenital malformations is more clearly understood. The possibility that intrauterine events influence health in later life[5] enhances the importance of pregnancy as a key target.

Prevention

Reports of the confidential enquiries into maternal deaths are always accompanied by detailed recommendations for service organisation, which are generally believed to have contributed to the fall in death rates. However, adherence to the recommendations is not universal. The effectiveness of interventions to prevent morbidity in the mother, from urinary tract infection to perineal pain after parturition, has now been explored by meta-analysis of all published

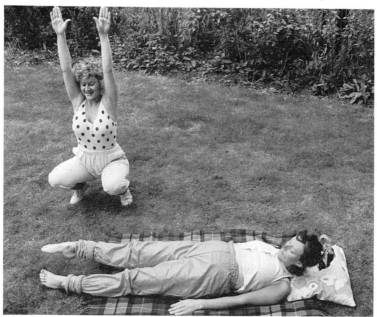

Adopting a healthy lifestyle is one way to improve health in pregnant women and their babies

and unpublished randomised controlled trials,[6] and a great many effective interventions are now known to be available. Alleviation of parental distress after miscarriage[7] and perinatal death[8] has been studied in different ways and much is known about how to address the problem. Prevention of unwanted pregnancy is a valid objective of family planning services, and there is some evidence about which types of service are most useful.[9]

Prevention of perinatal mortality and morbidity are usually considered together. Randomised controlled trials have found few effective interventions, perhaps because death is so uncommon and measures of morbidity hard to find. Some successful interventions are tight control of diabetes, cervical cerclage, and corticosteroids before preterm delivery, and many more interventions are known to reduce the rate of intermediate outcomes such as preterm delivery or low birth weight. Prevention of congenital malformation usually takes the form of averting the birth of the affected fetus by terminating pregnancy, but avoidance of teratogens and genetic counselling when appropriate can also have a useful impact.

Case against

The decline in maternal mortality has already been disproportionately large, so that maternal deaths form a lower proportion of all deaths of women in the reproductive age group than they did 30 years ago.[1] Study of avoidable death in the European Community[10] shows the United Kingdom in a less unfavourable light in respect of perinatal and maternal mortality than in respect of mortality from several other conditions, which suggests that there may be less scope for further intervention in perinatal and maternal mortality. Similarly, as the British induced abortion rate is among the lowest in the developed world, and as all methods of contraception have a recognised failure rate, it may be difficult to achieve any large reduction in unwanted pregnancy.

Perhaps the most cogent argument against regarding the health of pregnant women as a key target for the health strategy is that poor health is largely caused by social conditions. Gradients in perinatal mortality rates with social class[3 11] and other measures of deprivation[12] suggest that resources should be directed towards alleviation of poverty, poor housing, and malnutrition and curtailment of advertising of harmful substances such as alcohol and tobacco rather than towards health services. This of course may apply to other causes of ill health but is especially important in reproduction, partly because its success may be determined largely by events long before the pregnancy itself and because poverty may be precipitated by pregnancy, especially among single unsupported women, who often lose earnings and have special housing needs.

Possible targets

Perfect health for pregnant women cannot be an aim as improvements in care increasingly allow women with serious chronic diseases to try to have children. Choosing numerical targets at a national level may result in them proving unattainable for some health authorities but not particularly challenging for others because of large differences in existing levels of health and of service provision. Nevertheless, locally based targets for the health of pregnant women can be identified.

Most pregnancies should be wanted, which often, but not always, means they should be planned. Given the health problems of contraception,[13] however, the appropriate level of contraceptive use is for women to decide, and a target could be to make sure that all older school children are fully informed. Because counselling in unplanned pregnancy should be non-directive, no specific termination rate can be a target, but consumer surveys could assess the quality of counselling.

Ectopic pregnancy should be diagnosed as early as possible—Modern techniques allow the identification of almost every case before catastrophic haemorrhage occurs, and this is a realistic aim.

Miscarriage is not usually preventable, but it is important for psychological health that appropriate investigation and counselling should be offered, together with rubella immunisation of those negative for the antibody and treatment with anti-D immunoglobulin when appropriate.

Prenatal diagnosis—Though the cost effectiveness of screening programmes is important, the aim of the programme should not be to minimise the number of births of handicapped children but to offer reproductive choice to parents, provided resources are available. Thus the aim would be to offer full information to all parents eligible for screening to ensure that they had genuine choice and adequate support during periods of stress such as waiting for results or during and after termination or birth. Targets could be set for technical aspects of screening, such as good quality control on assays and tests, low rates of false positive and false negative results, and minimisation of morbidity after procedures, by adequate training.

Appropriate use of technology—New technology should not be widely used before it has been fully evaluated, but there is considerable doubt whether this is the case in respect of current practice of ultrasonography[14] or caesarean section.[3] Devolution of responsibility to primary care may reduce inappropriate use of technology, but this requires further evaluation.

Strategy for targets

The strategy for addressing the above and other goals could be based on the proposals of Banta[15]—for example, contracts specifying that all programmes of care to be purchased should be of proved efficacy, safety, and value. It is unlikely that this could be implemented immediately as there is often no consensus about what constitutes proof, but purchasers certainly ought to be discussing those matters. Because of women's overwhelming need and desire to have care and deliver as locally as possible, it is not practicable except in large urban areas to "shop around" for care, and outreach or devolution of care must be encouraged. Women's views of what are important health outcomes and services must be ascertained by surveys and discussion with consumer groups and incorporated in the strategy; they may well illustrate the "myth of infinite demand"[16] as many women prefer minimal intervention.

A prerequisite for meeting goals is investment in information systems. Some standardisation is needed for collection of data on critical matters such as classification of the cause of perinatal death, the lower gestation limit at which death is classified, indications for caesarean section, etc.

Problems in achieving targets

It will be difficult to make any valid assessment of whether targets are being achieved (because of poor routine data collection and doubt about whether rates of mortality and morbidity are population based) and not being distorted by selective referral and case mix differences. Targets may conflict—for example, the wish to reduce birth asphyxia might be thought to be incompatible with lowering the caesarean section rate, and fear of litigation may motivate the obstetrician. The proper aspirations of one set of health professionals may conflict with those of another—for example, midwives and general practitioners are both expert in the care of women with normal pregnancies. Financial considerations may interfere with appropriate tertiary referral. Planning and cooperation are more likely to promote better health than the competition which is proposed.

It may be difficult to quantify "soft" outcomes such as women's perceptions of counselling and grieving after bereavement without intrusive inquiries. Long term outcomes such as the birth or survival of children with handicaps may have implications for other public and private sectors and for families but may be invisible to those purchasing health care. Full health and economic assessment of strategies for intervention is essential.

Conclusion

Promotion of good health and nutrition in childhood will improve maternal health, but pregnancy is not too late for useful intervention, and failure to provide will mean paying a heavy price in terms of the health of future generations.

1 Confidential Enquiry into Maternal Deaths. *Report on the United Kingdom, 1985-7*. London: HMSO, 1991.
2 Kline J, Stein Z. The epidemiology of spontaneous abortion. In: Huisjes HJ, Lind T, eds. *Early pregnancy failure*. Edinburgh: Churchill Livingstone, 1990:240-56.
3 MacFarlane A, Mugford M. *Birth counts*. London: HMSO, 1984.
4 Bryce R, Stanley FJ, Blair E. The effects of intrapartum care on the risk of impairments in childhood. In: Chalmers I, Enkin M, Keirse MJNC, eds. *Effective care in pregnancy and childbirth*. Oxford: Oxford University Press, 1989:1313-21.
5 Barker DJP, Bull AR, Osmond C, Simmonds SJ. Fetal and placental size and risk of hypertension in adult life. *BMJ* 1990;**301**:259-62.
6 Chalmers I, Enkin M, Keirse MJNC, eds. *Effective care in pregnancy and childbirth*. Oxford: Oxford University Press, 1989.
7 Oakley A, McPherson A, Roberts H. *Miscarriage*. London: Penguin Books, 1990.
8 Forrest GC, Standish E, Baum JD. Support after a perinatal death: a study of support and counselling after perinatal bereavement. *BMJ* 1982;**285**: 1475-9.
9 Francome C. *Abortion practice in Britain and the United States*. London: Allen and Unwin, 1986.
10 Holland WW. *European Community atlas of avoidable death*. Oxford: Oxford University Press, 1988.
11 Townsend P, Davidson N, Whitehead M. *Inequalities in health: the Black report and the health divide*. London: Penguin, 1989.
12 Carstairs V, Morris R. *Deprivation and health in Scotland*. Aberdeen: Aberdeen University Press, 1991.
13 Beral V. Reproductive mortality. *BMJ* 1979;ii:632-4.
14 Temmerman M, Buekens P. Cost effectiveness of routine ultrasound examination in first trimester of pregnancy. *Eur J Obstet Gynecol Reprod Biol* 1991;**39**:13-8.
15 Banta D. National strategies for promoting effective care. In: Chalmers I, Enkin M, Keirse MJNC, eds. *Effective care in pregnancy and childbirth*. Oxford: Oxford University Press, 1989:1449-57.
16 Frankel S. Health needs, health care requirements and the myth of infinite demand. *Lancet* 1991;**337**:1588-90.

Accident prevention

I B PLESS

HAROLD BRIDGES LIBRARY
S. MARTIN'S COLLEGE
LANCASTER

The consultative document offers what is described as a new approach to improving the health of the population.[1] To an outsider it seems long overdue. There is an urgent need for such an initiative in general, but especially for accidents, which remain at epidemic levels. As Mr Waldegrave points out in his foreward, the need arises because the government's recent preoccupation with the management of the National Health Service is but one indirect way to meet the nation's health needs. To do so properly other more sweeping reforms are needed, especially those that decidedly shift the emphasis from medical care alone to at least equal investment in public health.

Should accidents be a key area?

The inclusion of accident reduction among the key areas is fully justified because it meets each of the specified criteria: injuries are a major cause of concern, there is wide scope for reducing them, and targets may easily be set.

Accidents are the leading cause of death among those under 30 and account for a greater proportion of years of potential life lost than cancer and heart disease combined.[2] They should also be a dominant concern because of the enormous costs to the NHS for treatment and rehabilitation.

The scope for improvement is especially compelling. A large number of proved measures await widespread implementation.[3] If there were similarly convincing evidence that equally effective means of preventing or treating cancer were available but not being implemented there would be a public outcry.

Finally, setting targets for accident reduction is easy—perhaps too

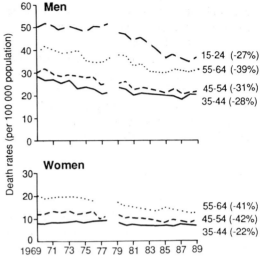

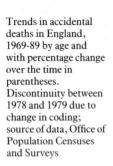

Trends in accidental deaths in England, 1969-89 by age and with percentage change over the time in parentheses. Discontinuity between 1978 and 1979 due to change in coding; source of data, Office of Population Censuses and Surveys

easy when they reflect only aggregate figures. Although any of several global rates can be chosen, because of what is known about the epidemiological patterns of injury such figures are much less meaningful than age and cause specific targets.

With a combination of these three criteria a convincing case could even be made for placing injury reduction at the very top of the list of key areas.

The case against

The very use of the term accidents may imply that accidents are random events, beyond human control. This notion, however, is entirely discredited. A large body of evidence convincingly shows that injuries are predictable and subject to the same rules of inquiry as any other scientific discipline.[4-7] The persistent use of "accident" in place of "injury,"[2] however, probably reinforces the pervasive view that injuries are largely inevitable.[8] Such a view, when held by policy makers, creates formidable barriers to progress.

In addition, because injuries are non-medical in that they are not prevented by the use of vaccines or treated by drugs they could be thought to have no place in a health document. This is, of course, nonsense. Treating the consequences of injuries entails a heavy expenditure of NHS resources, and the fact that prevention is largely accomplished by physical and social engineering is little different from the strategies used so effectively in preventing cholera, tuberculosis, and malnutrition.

Finally, some might argue that because at least six other central government departments, as well as local government, industry, commerce, and the voluntary sector, are concerned with accidents, accident prevention is only marginally a health matter. On the contrary, this diffusion of effort serves to underscore the tremendous need for strong leadership and adequate coordination.

Specifying targets

The target chosen for the year 2000 is a reduction in deaths due to accidents by at least 25% (box). As a decline greater than this occurred between 1980 and 1988 in people aged 55-64, this target seems reasonable. When, however, international data on children are compared the rates in 1985 in England were nearly twice those in Sweden.[9] Thus, based on the secretary of state's view that "international comparisons indicate the possibility for improvement," it is entirely reasonable to aim for much larger reductions—about half.

But setting one target for all age groups and for all types of injuries is misleading. The epidemiology of these events is such that far greater improvements can be made in some age groups and for some injuries than for others. Each should be targeted accordingly. For example, if the wearing of bicycle helmets were as widespread in England as in Victoria, Australia,[10] and if recent data from the US about their efficacy were applied,[11] a reduction in mortality from head injuries by about three quarters in a short time would be reasonable to expect. Conversely, some proved safety measures are less age specific—for example, requiring the universal use of smoke detectors or cracking down forcefully on drink-driving and on speeding violations.

The use of a global target is also mischievous because the multifaceted case of injury prevention results in responsibilities being widely diffused. It is then all too easy to imagine one department blaming another for failure to achieve the objective.

Strategies for reaching the targets

The best general strategy for reaching the target is not, as the document suggests, a matter of "in the end, increased awareness and

The government welcomes views on targets that might usefully be set in accident prevention:

- Should the targets look only as far as the year 2000 or would long term development be better served by looking beyond that date?
- The World Health Organisation European target for accidents is that by the year 2000 death from accidents should be reduced by at least 25% from 1980 values through an intensified effort to reduce traffic, house, and occupational accidents. The indicator for this target is mortality. What scope is there for using other indicators, such as measures of temporary or permanent injury and morbidity—for example, long absence from work, and length of stay in hospital?
- Should targets be for the population generally, or for specific groups—for example, children and elderly people—or should both approaches be used?

carefulness of individuals." It might be if these behaviours were readily modified, but this cannot be brought simply by education and persuasion alone. Instead the changes needed will require the other forms of action listed in the document: legislation, improved engineering and design, and improvements in living and working environments.

Furthermore, it is only half true to suggest that because "the range of those with the opportunity to contribute is . . . wide . . . accident prevention is *par excellence* an example of an area where the best results are achieved by cooperation and collaboration." Cooperation will work well only if the Department of Health accepts full responsibility for ensuring that the agreed goals are achieved. Although voluntary cooperation—for example, by the public—is clearly preferable, regulation, legislation, and other forms of coercion are usually more effective. Ideally, however, such steps should be taken only when the public accepts that they are necessary and wise; educational techniques serve well in this sort of pump priming operation.

One obstacle in determining strategies for reaching the target is the fact that the consultative document gives the appearance of having done too little homework. In similar preliminary documents produced by the US surgeons general, goals are specified in much greater detail; they reflect widespread consultation; and they are based on a thorough review of existing knowledge and current statistics.[12]

Problems in achieving the targets

As matters now stand, despite the document's many good intentions the target for accidents is unlikely to be achieved. This is because the time span is too short; there is no assurance that sufficient resources will be made available; and, above all, there is little indication that the Department of Health intends to fight the political battles that will need to be fought to achieve sufficient resources and control. Not seeking such leadership and not establishing mechanisms for truly effective coordination are tantamount to an admission of defeat.

Consider two current examples. Road accidents are the largest cause of deaths from injury yet they remain chiefly the responsibility of the Department of Transport. At a recent launch of a bicycle helmet promotion campaign the Department of Health was not even represented. Similarly, it was silent when an attempt to include random breath testing in the new road traffic bill failed. This occurred in spite of cross party support for the motion, endorsement by the Parliamentary Advisory Council for Transport Safety and the BMA, and the indisputable public health importance of this measure. Instead, the government, prompted by the Home Office, imposed a three line whip to defeat the motion. Would the new department argue vigorously that in doing so its mandate and mission were being thwarted? If not, what meaning lies behind the high sounding rhetoric about accepting responsibility? Are future transport ministers to have the final say on such matters, arguing as Mr Chope, under secretary of state, has done, that striking the right balance between the need for effective enforcement of the law and the freedom of the individual is paramount, even when public health is involved?

The Department of Health must assume ultimate responsibility because the Department of Transport, and indeed all other government departments, have other interests to serve and other goals to meet. Only the Department of Health is influenced exclusively by health considerations. Hence a major problem in achieving a significant reduction is that the Department of Health seems not to be convinced that accident prevention lies within its sphere of interest. If it were the action plan described in the report of the National

Association of Health Authorities and Royal Society for the Prevention of Accidents Strategy Group would be in the process of implementation, but it is not.[13]

It also seems that no thought has been given to creating within the Department of Health a structure similar to the Division of Injury Control in the US, which now seems essential to success in accident prevention.

Conclusion

If injuries are health problems—and because they result in death, pain, suffering, disability, or disfigurement they surely are—all key elements essential to their control must fall predominantly within the aegis of the health department. Regrettably, the document does not accept such a responsibility, nor does it give any indication that steps will be taken to affirm that in accident prevention, and indeed in all health matters, the Department of Health is first among equals.

The secretary of state wisely underscores the key role health authorities ought to have in maintaining and improving health, and elsewhere the document acknowledges that they have, in part, failed to perform this task adequately. The reasons for this are numerous and too well known to merit repetition. To address public health issues properly necessitates going beyond concerns about the NHS, requiring as well a fundamental shift in the philosophy of the Department of Health. Ironically, the document makes such a commitment: the secretary of state states that the department's task is "to *take the action necessary, or ensure that . . . action is taken*, whether through the NHS or otherwise, to improve and protect health" (my italics). This underscores the view that in the end responsibility for accident prevention lies with the department, whether or not the NHS is directly involved. This position is, as Mr Waldegrave points out, fully in line with other major historical events in public health and hence not as radical as it may at first seem. Furthermore, although, as has been stated, many other bodies have a role in accident prevention, to be effective they must be properly coordinated, and for the Department of Health to do this is a large departure from past and current practice.

Without such measures the aim of "restoring the balance between prevention, treatment and rehabilitation" is doomed. Placing greater emphasis on prevention is by no means misplaced, nor is it wrong to seek to change behaviour to promote health. The secretary of state mistakenly seems to believe that techniques for behavioural change are well developed. They are not, and until they improve greatly the balance between the role of individual people and that of government must inevitably be with the government. He further assumes that simply providing the necessary information will lead to wise, free choices and that accordingly "education is the key." This is a naive, Utopian dream that may some day come true, but not, as matters now stand, in the near future.[14]

It is easy to think that there will be no coherent preventive health programme until after the next election. But it is not just the fiddling about and the delay that should be of concern. The proposed reforms do not go far enough. The central question of how much responsibility the department wishes to assume to ensure that its objectives are met remains elusive, especially in the case of accident prevention. Perhaps this is deliberate. The issue is engulfed in a web of ambiguity and waffle. On the one hand, the document takes many of the right positions; on the other, it is far from evident that the department intends to take the steps needed to ensure that it has the power to achieve these stout intentions. To do so the tools and resources that go with central responsibility must be sharper and more powerful than any alluded to in this document.

1 Secretary of State for Health. *The health of the nation.* London: HMSO, 1991.
2 The National Committee for Injury Prevention and Control. Injury prevention: meeting the challenge. *Am J Prev Med* 1989;5:5-6.
3 Rivara FP. Epidemiology of childhood injuries. I. Review of current research and presentation of conceptual framework. *Am J Dis Child* 1982;**136**:399-405.
4 Haddon W. Advances in the epidemiology of injuries as a basis for public policy. *Public Health Rep* 1980;**95**:411-21.
5 Robertson LS. *Injuries: causes, control strategies, and public policy.* Lexington, Massachusetts: Lexington Books, 1983.
6 Waller JA. *Injury control: a guide to the causes and prevention of trauma.* Lexington, Massachusetts: Lexington Books, 1985.
7 Baker SP, O'Neill B, Karpf RS. *The injury fact book.* Lexington, Massachusetts: Lexington Books, 1984.
8 Langley JD. The need to discontinue the use of the term "accident" when referring to unintentional injury events. *Accident Analysis and Prevention* 1988;**20**:1-8.
9 Fingerhutt L, Kleinman J. Trends and current status in childhood mortality, United States, 1900-1985. *Vital Health Stat* 1989;**26**:1-44.
10 McDermott FT. Helmets for bicyclists—another first for Victoria. *Med J Aust* 1991;**154**:156-7.
11 Thompson RS, Rivara FP, Thompson DC. A case-control study of the effectiveness of bicycle safety helmets. *N Engl J Med* 1989;**320**:1361-7.
12 US Department of Health, Education and Welfare. *Healthy people: the surgeon general's report on health promotion and disease prevention.* Washington, DC: DHEW, 1979. (DHEW Publication No (PHS) 79-55071A.)
13 National Association of Health Authorities—Royal Society for the Prevention of Accidents Strategy Group. *Report. Action on accidents: the unique role of the health service.* Birmingham: NAHA, 1990.
14 Pless IB, Arsenault L. The role of health education in the prevention of injuries to children. *Journal of Social Issues* 1987;**43**:87-103.

Children's health

DAVID HULL

The main theme of *The Health of the Nation*[1] is the prevention of ill health and the promotion of good health. One of the suggested key areas is the health of pregnant women, infants, and children. I have been asked to consider the health of infants and children and to discuss what if any are the appropriate targets and how they should be met.

Selection as key area

The consultative document proposes three criteria for the selection of key areas: the areas should be a major cause of premature death or avoidable ill health, effective interventions should be possible, and it should be possible to set objectives and targets. On this basis there is ample justification for including child health as a key area.

The key areas proposed do not have like characteristics; some are concerned with avoiding diseases or their effects (such as asthma) and others with avoiding hazards (such as accident prevention). All the areas are as relevant to children as they are to adults, indeed in many instances, more so. Strategies for disease prevention are likely to have most impact in childhood and the risks of the hazards to health are often greater in the vulnerable years. The benefits of a clean safe environment, immunisation programmes, a healthy diet, avoidance of accidents, pyschological wellbeing, etc are more likely to be greater and last longer when applied to infants and children. The health of children is not only an area it is central to the whole strategy, and so it seems inappropriate to isolate parts of it for specific targets.

Can the government deliver, and if it cannot will it do more harm than good to be identified as a key area? Over the years the government has issued documents urging health promotion and sickness prevention without clear directions on how their recommendations should be implemented. To succeed the strategy has to be central to all health service activities—primary, secondary, and tertiary; health promotion should not be the responsibility solely of enthusiasts with little or no clinical responsibility. The cardiac

---

Possibilities for improving child health and targets in the green paper

The scope for safeguarding and improving children's health includes:

(i) For younger children
- Immunisation against childhood disease
- Early detection of congenital and acquired abnormalities including impairments in hearing, vision, growth, and development

(ii) For older children
- Promotion of healthy lifestyle
- Prevention (particularly through education) of smoking and misuse of alcohol and drugs

(iii) For all children
- Accident prevention and safety education
- Improvements in the quality of the environment, particularly housing
- Avoidance of smoking in the household
- Prevention, identification, and treatment of emotional and behavioural problems
- Prevention of dental decay

Targets:

To increase nationally the proportion of infants who are breast fed at birth from 64% in 1985 to 75% by 2000.

To increase nationally the proportion of infants aged 6 weeks being wholly or partly breast fed from 39% in 1985 to 50% by 2000.

By 2003, nationally, 12 year olds should on average have no more than 1·5 decayed, missing, or filled permanent teeth.

---

surgeon should aim at avoiding the need to operate, not at being rewarded for increasing trade.

The authors of the strategy are optimistic because of the opportunities presented by the NHS reforms and the release of the Department of Health from day to day management of services. That suggests a confidence in the future which those of us who see patients would like to share. It was the reformers of 1974 who failed to appreciate the importance of the public health function and planned the contraction of the child health and school medical services, whose primary tasks were precisely those outlined in this new document. Nevertheless, children's doctors have every reason to be optimists and tend to trust those in authority, and we would all like to see the government succeed in this initiative.

Appropriate targets

Though the overall objectives for the health of infants and children are in general admirable, the three proposed targets are weak (box). Two are concerned with breast feeding. There was a welcome increase

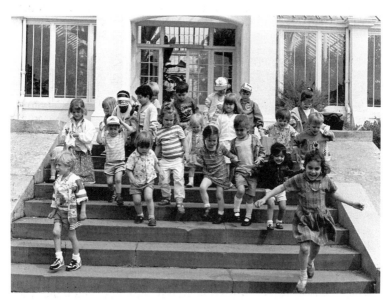

Strategies to promote health are likely to have more impact in children

in the rate of breast feeding during 1970-80[2] but there has been little sign of increase since; if anything there has been a slight fall. I doubt this reflects mothers' ignorance of the relative merits of breast and bottle feeding but rather social attitudes and expectations. Given the social conditions of our times some might challenge the net benefit of higher rates of breast feeding. The rate of breast feeding in Hong Kong is much lower than that in Britain, but their overall health statistics are better. If health statistics depend on economic success and if economic success depends on two income families then it is employers who can do most to improve the rate of breast feeding. An alternative target might be to reduce the percentage of mothers who express a wish or intention to breast feed on booking for pregnancy care who fail to do so. It is to be hoped that the current breast feeding initiative will succeed and the government's targets will be reached long before the year 2000.

The third target relating to children is to reduce dental caries. This is already a considerable success story, and it is both reasonable and desirable to expect more.

Thus little in these three targets challenges the paediatric and the child health services or the other authorities and departments whose activities affect the health of children. For this reason I wish to suggest some new target areas. The areas are only a sample, and I could suggest many more.

Premature birth

A major cause of neonatal (and therefore infant) death is premature birth. In Nottingham neonatal mortality in babies born before 32 weeks' gestation has improved little over the past 10 years. The rate compares favourably with that in other countries whereas total neonatal mortality, though comparable with the national figure, is above that in some European countries, Japan, and Hong Kong, mainly because we have a higher incidence of premature births. Only 10% of neonatal deaths are in infants over 32 weeks' gestation without lethal congenital anomalies. One target could be to reduce the numbers of preterm births. The percentage of low birthweight infants is one of eight measures used by the Center for the Study of Social Policy in the US for comparing the wellbeing of children in different states. As a target it would have more to recommend it than mortality alone, for if the rate of preterm birth was reduced mortality and morbidity would fall whereas reducing only mortality might increase morbidity.

Preterm births, however, would be only a long distance measure of child health services and are perhaps more directly an outcome of obstetric care. The strategy document argues that geographic, age group, and social class differences are strong gounds for believing that there are remedial causative factors. Therefore, an alternative target would be to reduce the variation in the numbers of preterm births.

Surveillance programmes

It is important that we learn from the success of the vaccination programme in the past 10 years. In my view success is attributable to two factors. Firstly, there is a strong central leadership which has moved from a permissive stance to actively promoting the programme, exploring the reasons why it was failing, identifying both general and local factors, and addressing them directly and, secondly, a network has been established across the health districts, with doctors identified in each health authority to be responsible for promoting the service.

The same framework is being established for child health surveillance programmes, and they should be given targets within the national strategy. One aim could be the identification of children with poor growth in the first year of life, with a target to reduce the number of children below a certain size at 1 year of age. There is some evidence that poor weight gain in the first year of life is associated with early death from heart disease. Another could be the incidence of iron deficiency anaemia. Chronic iron deficiency is associated with poor performance at school. A third could be the identification of all children in a district with a severe disability (physical, mental, hearing, vision) and to set a target to reduce the incidence over five years and to reduce the difference between the social groups. These tasks would not be that exacting as they are central to any surveillance strategy, but the remedies would require a multidisciplinary programme.

Child care and protection

Family break up is increasing and it is occurring when the children are younger.[3] Child care and protection are making increasing demands on many services, including the health service. Homelessness and misery in adolescence also seem to be increasing. It should be possible to identify targets in these areas—for example, that the health of children in care should be equal to that of those who are not (for example, vaccination rates) and that the numbers of adolescents who suffer for want of a sensitive service should be reduced to a minimum, as indicated, for example, by the rates of teenage pregnancies, suicides, or drug misuse.

To meet the green paper requirements a target must be important, avoidable, and measurable. This means that many important problems will be overlooked. I can seen no reason why a marker of the problem—for example, teenage pregnancies—cannot be used as a pointer to the health care of adolescents. It would of course require that the association between the marker target and the problem was explored.

Meeting the targets

It would be impossible to do more than outline the strategies needed to address the new targets I have proposed. They all depend on establishing a comprehensive, coordinated paediatric and child health service in every health district. The interface between this support service and the family practitioner service must be clearly defined. Clear central guidance would be needed on priorities and data collection, with informed analysis within each health authority. Success will depend on the wholehearted, informed cooperation of parents; parent held records are a first but important step in enabling parents to share in promoting the health of the nation's children.

It is not difficult to think of reasons why an initiative like this might not succeed. It is essential that the slimmed down Department of Health when it announces its priorities acknowledges that those not included are left out because of resource limitations. It would be wrong and unrealistic to expect doctors and other health professionals to strive to achieve higher and higher standards within their duty to care and to chase centrally set targets without giving them extra resources. The exercise is central to all health service activities and it should therefore be implemented through contracts between health authorities and provider units, all provider units. Even so it will be important to engage the new managers in the spirit of the exercise.

It was encouraging to read the section in the green paper giving the contribution of other government departments to the health of the nation. Many of the initiatives will fail without some requirement that the various departments act together. With respect to child health, there must be local arrangements that ensure the departments of health, social services, and education and local authorities cooperate rather than compete. There has been little success in recent memory.

Just look at the special needs registers of the different authorities.

My last concern is one that continually taxes paediatricians in neonatal intensive care: Will we ever be able to adopt a health care policy that admits it cannot afford the most recent expensive high tech approach and that chooses to take a long term, "green" view of its responsibilities?

Closing comment

One of the criteria for a target area is that it can be measured. Quality caring rather than quality care is not easily measured, but it is what patients want. Caring will always depend on the dedication and the professionalism of the staff. The document identifies a "highly dedicated and professional workforce" as one of the strengths of the NHS. That, in no small measure, reflects the education and inspiration provided by those who teach, an aspect of our service in Britain that must not be overlooked in our desire to set clinical standards and outcome measures and desirable targets that can be measured.

1 Secretary of State for Health. *The Health of the Nation.* London: HMSO, 1991. (Cm 1523.)
2 Department of Health and Social Security, Child Nutrition Panel of Committee on Medical Aspects of Food Policy. *Present day practice in infant feeding. Third report.* London: HMSO, 1988.
3 Central Statistical Office. *Social Trends No 21.* London: HMSO, 1991.

Cancer

C J WILLIAMS

The Health of the Nation is a wide ranging consultative document.[1] Though reduction in cancer mortality and morbidity is included as a suggested key objective, only limited aims are included in the section on objectives and targets for action. This is somewhat surprising as cancer is the second leading cause of death and causes more lost years of life than any other disease in Britain.[2] Indeed, as the document makes clear, England has the highest mortality from cancer among the industrialised countries. Thus cancer fulfils the first of the criteria by which the document judges the key areas—it is a major health problem.

One of the problems with cancer is that it is often thought of as a single condition. Only when viewed as individual tumour entities do some types of cancer achieve the second of the government's criteria for key areas—namely, that effective interventions are possible. The specific targets for cancer identified in the document are shown in the box. Only the targets relating to breast and cervical cancers are mentioned specifically in the section on cancer, though there is clearly an overlap with other topics covered in the document, particularly smoking.

Scope for breast and cervical cancer

The scope of the objectives for breast and cervical cancer contrasts bizarrely. It seems laudable, though optimistic, to expect in a national population a 25% reduction in deaths from breast cancer during a 10 year period when some research workers doubt the effectiveness of screening[3 4] and when some randomised trials and case-control studies have failed to identify such a large benefit in a similar population.[5 6] In

71

Government's targets for cancer

- To reduce deaths from breast cancer in women aged 50-64 (the group invited for mammographic screening) by 25% by the year 2000 compared with 1990 values
- To invite all women aged 20-64 for cervical screening by the end of 1993
- To reduce the prevalence of smoking to 22% in men and 21% in women (reductions of 33% and 30% respectively) by the year 2000. This target for cancers associated with smoking is mentioned specifically in the annex on smoking

support of the document's aims two overviews suggest that such a reduction in mortality is possible.[7][8] It is too early to assess what has been achieved in Britain, but in 1988 the UK Trial of Early Detection of Breast Cancer Group reported the results of mammography every other year in 45 841 women.[5] A further 63 636 women were offered teaching of breast self examination, and there was a comparison group of 127 117 women for whom no extra services were provided. These cohorts of women were enrolled between 1979 and 1981. Mortality was reduced in the women screened by mammography. The unadjusted reduction was 14% (relative risk 0·86%, 95% confidence interval 0·69 to 1·08) and even when other factors were adjusted for the reduction in mortality did not reach conventional significance. The reputation of the two screening districts (Edinburgh and Guildford) is high and such skill in breast screening is not available nationally. The acceptance rates of 60% and 72% in Edinburgh and Guildford, respectively, may not be achieved in the long term in a national programme, although it is encouraging that breast cancer is primarily a disease of middle class women and that breast cancer rates among non-acceptors in some studies are lower than those among acceptors.[9] The authors of this paper emphasise, however, the need for high acceptance rates and high sensitivity of screening (with a likely loss of specificity) if targets are to be achieved. Whether the target can be achieved remains to be seen, but even a 10-15% reduction in mortality is likely to be worth while.

In contrast to its target for breast cancer, all the government suggests for cervical cancer is that all eligible women be invited for screening. As non-attenders are those at greatest risk,[10] a much more

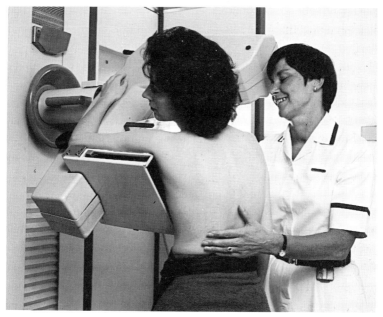

Though the government's target for reducing deaths from breast cancer might not be achievable, even a 10-15% reduction in mortality would be worth while

vigorous campaign is required if it is to have an impact on survival — the simple aim that all women be invited is likely to achieve a political target without significantly affecting mortality.

Scope for other cancers

Early detection of cancer has been called into doubt,[11] and its clinical significance pales in comparison with the impact of reducing smoking, which is included as a separate key area. Achievement of the government's aim, reduction in smoking rates to 22% for men and 21% for women by the year 2000, is bound to reduce mortality from lung cancer as well as that from several other smoking related cancers. In addition, the reduction in the risk of cardiovascular and respiratory diseases is an important bonus. Nearly all commentators will agree that reduced cigarette smoking should be the prime aim of any health programme for the nation. With these targets in mind, however, it seems overambitious to rely so heavily on the effects of education. Although previous educational programmes have been effective in reducing smoking, further attempts are likely to suffer from the law of

73

diminishing returns and may succeed simply in reinforcing the present level of consumption. This one key area is the acid test of the government's will to improve the nation's health. Whether it will grasp the nettle and progressively increase cigarette prices and taxation and reduce the amount of advertising and sponsorship are open to question. Only when this government introduces progressive policies on taxation and advertising for smoking will the nation be convinced that disease prevention is high on its political agenda.

The section on diet also overlaps with cancer—in their monograph on the causes of cancer, Peto and Doll rate diet alongside smoking as a major cause of this disease.[12] Data are, however, insufficient to recommend a specific diet. The rather bland assertion in *The Health of the Nation* to reduce the intake of saturated fatty acids and total fat together with reducing obesity rates and excessive alcohol consumption may well have some effect on cancer. Several common malignancies, such as breast cancer, are directly correlated with increasing obesity,[13] and a reduction in fat intake and consequent obesity may reduce the risk of some tumours. Similarly, cancers of the mouth, throat, larynx, and oesophagus are closely correlated with high alcohol intake and there is a synergistic relation with smoking.[14] However, though many people may understand this and wish to change their (and their families') diet, financial constraints may prevent it. If this happens we may end up blaming the victim.

Other indirect gains may come from other key areas. These include HIV infection and AIDS (there are no specific targets included), in which changes in sexual habits and the increased use of condoms may reduce the risk of cervical cancer if recent theories on viral aetiology are correct.[15] Similarly, reduced exposure to environmental carcinogens may be beneficial—though Peto and Doll estimate that such exposure accounts for less than 5% of all cancers in the United States.[12]

Conclusions

Overall, *The Health of the Nation* is an encouraging document in that it tries to identify the key problems, asks whether there are means for improvement, and then targets objectives. However, the consultation process will need to greatly strengthen what is currently an anodyne document. Though successful screening for breast and cervical cancers are attractive goals, they are far less cost effective than reducing the rate of smoking. Although the document talks about treatment, rehabilitation, and counselling in other key areas, there is little mention of these topics in relation to cancer. Targets could easily be set in terms of providing information, training medical and nurse specialists (staffing in Britain is far below that in other industrialised countries), and providing counselling services and rehabilitation facilities. By focusing on two issues, that the public believes are important (screening for breast and cervical cancer) the government is in danger of merely tinkering with the problem. Above all else, it should make clear that it is willing to reduce smoking through legislative means. Only then are screening, diet, information, and counselling kept in proportion. In addition, the government has the machinery, the resources, and the infrastructure to deliver high quality care to those who need it. Improvements in survival and quality of life are likely to be achieved when all of these measures are implemented.

1 Secretary of State for Health. *The health of the nation*. London: HMSO, 1991.
2 Cancer Research Campaign. *Trends in cancer survival in Great Britain 1982*. London: CRC, 1982.
3 Rodgers A. Breast screening in women aged 65-79. *BMJ* 1991;**302**:411.
4 Roberts MM. Breast screening: time for a rethink? *BMJ* 1989;**299**:1153-5.
5 UK Trial of Early Detection of Breast Cancer Group. First results on mortality reduction in the UK trial of early detection of breast cancer. *Lancet* 1988;ii:41-6.
6 Andersson I, Aspegren K, Janzon L, Landberg T, Lindholm K, Linell F, *et al*. Mammographic screening and mortality from breast cancer: the Malmö mammographic screening trial. *BMJ* 1988;**297**:943-8.
7 Gray JAM. *Breast cancer screening 1991. Evidence and experience since the Forrest report*. Sheffield: Trent Regional Health Authority, 1991.
8 Wald N, Frost C, Cuckle H. Breast cancer screening: the current position. *BMJ* 1991;**302**: 845-6.
9 Fink K, Shapiro S, Lewison J. The reluctant participant in a breast screening programme. *Public Health Rep* 1968;**63**:479-90.
10 Guzick DS. Efficacy of screening for cervical cancer: a review. *Am J Public Health* 1978;**68**: 125-34.
11 Skrabanek P. False premises and false promises of breast screening. *Lancet* 1985;ii:318-20.
12 Doll R, Peto R. *The causes of cancer*. Oxford: Oxford University Press, 1981.
13 Lew EA, Garfinkel L. Variations in mortality by weight among 750 000 men and women. *Journal of Chronic Diseases* 1979;**32**:563-76.
14 Tuyns AJ, Péquignot G, Jensen OM. Les cancers de l'oesophage en Ille-et-Villaine en fonction des niveaux de consommation d'alcool et de tabac. Des risques qui se multiplient. *Bull Cancer (Paris)* 1977;**64**:45-60.
15 Genital human papillomavirus infections. *American College of Obstetricians and Gynaecologists' Technical Bulletin* 1987;No 105.

Strategy for asthma

P G J BURNEY

The government's consultative document *The Health of the Nation* marks a clear change in focus for the Department of Health[1] away from the day to day issues of health service management towards a more active role in broader public health issues. Among its objectives it lists the reduction in deaths and ill health attributable to asthma, firstly, by the effective provision of health services and, in the long term, by establishing the aetiology of the disease.

Why asthma should be a key area

Asthma poses a major challenge to public health. Not only is it one of the commonest causes of chronic ill health but it is also an increasing problem. In childhood, asthma is the commonest cause of losing time from school[2] and has become one of the commonest causes of admission to hospital.[3] Information on exactly how much asthma restricts adults' activity is less easy to determine. The Department of Health estimates that among the working population seven million working days were lost because of asthma in 1987-8.[1]

Rates of admission to hospital,[4] prescribing,[5] and consultation in general practice[6] are all rising, and the evidence suggests that the prevalence of asthma is also increasing, at least among children.[7 8] These increases, which are probably due to an increasing incidence, are not confined to the United Kingdom but have been widely reported around the world. Mortality from asthma also rose in the late 1970s and early 1980s and has not declined since.[9] Whether this increase in mortality represents an increase in case fatality or simply reflects the change in prevalence is difficult to judge from the infor-

76

mation available. However, it is likely that at least some of the increase is attributable to the growing prevalence.[10]

On the current evidence asthma is a preventable disease. The rapid increase and wide variation in prevalence and the changes in prevalence noted among migrants suggest an environmental component in the aetiology of asthma, which should be reversible. If the adverse changes that have been noted are largely the result of a changing incidence, logic dictates that the thrust of any health strategy should be towards primary prevention of the disease.

It is also likely that asthma could be better managed. There are now effective drugs for managing asthma, including both anti-inflammatory drugs and bronchodilators. There are also agreed guidelines for the management of asthma in children[11] and in adults, both for long term treatment[12] and for acute exacerbations.[13] These guidelines are not yet widely followed, and shortcomings in the management of asthma have been reported to be associated with deaths from asthma,[14] patients admitted to hospital with asthma,[15] and children missing school because of asthma.[16]

Government's possible targets for asthma

● There are several difficulties in setting targets—firstly, the identification of the targets themselves, and, secondly, their quantification. Simple targets related to reductions in mortality will be difficult to set because the factors which lead to death are not sufficiently well understood. Targets should therefore concentrate initially on reducing the amount of avoidable ill health

● It may be best to develop targets for defined populations based on adherence to published clinical management guidelines, the establishment of agreed protocols between general practitioners and hospital clinicians, the development of district wide strategies, etc. Monitoring the uptake of peak flow meters on prescription and the development of self management plans may also offer some scope for developing targets

● Work will be necessary to establish the link between such measures and health outcome. Consultation between the government, the NHS, and other interested parties will be necessary to develop suitable targets

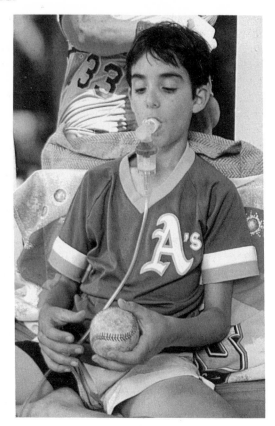

Reducing deaths and
ill health attributable
to asthma is a key
government objective

Case against

It is easy to argue that a reduction in morbidity from asthma should
be a principal objective of government policy, but the case for setting
targets is more difficult to argue and depends on how the targets are to
be used. *The Health of the Nation* is not clear on this point.[1] If targets
are set simply to give direction to a programme of work and to allow
progress to be monitored they do not pose great problems. If, on the
other hand, they are to be used more specifically to set incentives, as
with the recent changes to the general practitioners' contract, they
would raise much greater difficulties.

Firstly, there is a problem with the case definition of asthma.
Where specific surveillance systems can be set up this may not be an

issue as standardisation and consistency are more important than adherence to some as yet undefined gold standard. Prevalence has thus been monitored over the past 18 years in English primary schools by the national study of health and growth,[8] and as the condition is common it would be possible to include similar questions in other national surveillance programmes. But surveillance based on diagnosed asthma, particularly in general practice where labelling might be variable, is unlikely to be useful. Targets such as the proportion of asthmatic patients with peak flow meters or with agreed management plans would be strongly influenced by the level of diagnosis.

A second problem arises when setting targets relating to aspects of care about which some of the evidence is now controversial. The current debate over the use of inhaled β agonists is the most obvious example,[17] but this is not the only contentious issue. Inhaled steroids are now suspected of producing more systemic side effects than was previously believed,[18 19] and many of the procedures that are thought to be self evidently good remain unproved in practice. For instance, much of the evidence in England on the effects of health education[20] or self management[21 22] is unclear. Studies of self management have either been uncontrolled[21] or have shown no significant difference between active and control treatments.[22] In a condition such as asthma, which has a very variable course, this must lead to some reservations concerning the efficacy of these methods of controlling it, at least as tested.

These reservations should not be overinterpreted. There is at least evidence that respiratory physicians do better than general physicians in managing asthma.[23 24] This implies that current specialist practice has important advantages and supports the view that abandoning current methods of management is likely to have worse consequences than continuing their use.[25] Secondly, evidence on health education from the United States is more ambivalent, and some studies suggest that intensive programmes may be effective in reducing the numbers of emergency room visits[26] or hospital readmissions.[27] Whether this is due to a different message in the American health education, differences in the patients, or a difference in the medical environment is not clear. However, though some encouragement can be gained from these findings, they are not yet adequate to sustain specific claims for large amounts of resources or strong incentives for individual aspects of management.

The targets

As the principal problem with asthma is its increasing prevalence it is rational to set this as the main target to be monitored. Prevalence is currently monitored in primary school children,[8] and monitoring could be extended to other national surveys without much difficulty. Monitoring the loss of quality of life due to asthma could also provide evidence on the overall effectiveness of the health services. As asthma is common it is reasonable to believe that monitoring would be informative within the likely sample size of any national programme. It might also be possible to monitor absence from school due to asthma, though case definition would be a problem and surveillance would add another administrative burden to a hard pressed education service.

Potential targets that are already measured routinely are difficult to identify. Mortality should be a target but death from asthma is rare and short term changes in death rates are unreliable. Rates of admission to hospital are hard to interpret: high rates may indicate both inadequate control of the disease in the community and an appropriate response to uncontrolled disease. Incentives to reduce hospital admissions could have perverse effects if this were not taken into account and if appropriate referrals to hospital were discouraged. Intermediate targets could be set by assessing adherence to the current guidelines on the management of asthma. Use of these guidelines is currently limited by uncertainty over management and by difficulty, at least in general practice, over case definition.

Achieving the objective

Three things are essential if the current trends are to be reversed. Firstly, we need to understand why the prevalence of asthma is increasing. There are now several clues suggesting possible reasons, but a coordinated research programme is required to test these rigorously and develop a preventive strategy for asthma. All the evidence strongly suggests that asthma is predominantly an environmental disease and that the current trends could be reversed. If current trends in mortality, admission to hospital, consultations, and prescribing are largely determined by changes in prevalence then primary prevention is the only credible long term strategy for dealing with the underlying problem.

Secondly, a further programme of research is required into the effectiveness and safety of different methods of managing asthma. It would be naive to assume that a treatment regimen free of side effects is available, but recent controversies have shown up several weaknesses in the scientific basis for the current management of asthma. We need to know more about both the long term effects of treatment and the other factors that influence the adequate control of asthma. Even if all the current anxieties are shown to be without foundation the current uncertainty alone could reduce the number of people getting adequate treatment. Moreover, it will remain difficult to insist on a particular form of management without clear evidence that it is both effective and efficient.

In the meantime it is important that current guidelines[11-13] should be widely known and adhered to. They remain the best opinion that we have on the optimal management of asthma and such circumstantial evidence as we have suggests that patients treated according to these guidelines are likely to do better than those who are treated otherwise. Adherence to guidelines is probably best achieved through the organisation of local audit of asthma care.

Finally, it is necessary to inform the public more fully about what they should expect. Low expectations are probably as much a barrier to good management of asthma as any single defect in the health services.

Expected problems

The Health of the Nation indicates a change of emphasis towards more strategic issues.[1] Ironically, the section on asthma reverses this emphasis and focuses on managing the health services' response. Though there is clearly room for improvement in the way that asthma is managed, this reversal is unfortunate. If the principal problem is an increase in the prevalence and severity of asthma then this is the issue that should be addressed.

One problem with accepting a reduction in the prevalence and severity of asthma as a principal objective is that achieving it depends on a successful programme of research. While there is every prospect of this research being successful in the next few years such success cannot be taken for granted. Moreover, successful research is only the first requirement. Just as important is the application of the results of that research to an integrated programme for the prevention of asthma. For this to be successful it is important that the Department of Health should play an active part. Over the past decade almost all the initiatives have come from charities such as the National Asthma

Campaign and professional bodies such as the British Thoracic Society. The greatest barrier to achieving a lower prevalence of asthma would be the Department of Health failing to live up to the promise of *The Health of the Nation* and reverting to the view that only those problems that have simple managerial solutions are of relevance to its strategy.

1 Secretary of State for Health. *The Health of the Nation*. London: HMSO, 1991. (Cm 1523.)
2 Nocon A. Social and emotional impact of childhood asthma. *Arch Dis Child* 1991;**66**:458-60.
3 Hill AM. Trends in paediatric medical admissions. *BMJ* 1989;**298**:1479-83.
4 Alderson M. Trends in morbidity and mortality from asthma. *Population Trends* 1987;**49**:18-23.
5 Hay I, Higginbottam T. Has the management of asthma improved? *Lancet* 1987;i:609-11.
6 Fleming DM, Crombie DL. Prevalence of asthma and hay fever in England and Wales. *BMJ* 1987;**294**:279-83.
7 Burr ML, Butland BK, King S, Vaughan-Williams E. Changes in asthma prevalence: two surveys 15 years apart. *Arch Dis Child* 1989;**64**:1452-6.
8 Burney PGJ, Chinn S, Rona R. Has the prevalence of asthma increased in children? Evidence from the National Study of Health and Growth 1973-86. *BMJ* 1990;**300**:1306-10.
9 Burney PGJ. Asthma mortality in England and Wales: evidence for a further increase 1974-1984. *Lancet* 1986;ii:323-6.
10 Burney PGJ. Asthma deaths in England and Wales 1931-1985: evidence for a true increase in asthma mortality. *J Epidemiol Community Health* 1988;**42**: 316-20.
11 Warner JO, Götz M, Landon LI, Levison H, Milner AD, Pedersen S, *et al*. Management of asthma: a consensus statement. *Arch Dis Child* 1989;**64**: 165-79.
12 British Thoracic Society, Research Unit of Royal College of Physicians of London, King's Fund Centre, National Asthma Campaign. Guidelines for management of asthma in adults: I. Chronic persistent asthma. *BMJ* 1990;**301**:6513.
13 British Thoracic Society, Research Unit of Royal College of Physicians of London, King's Fund Centre, National Asthma Campaign. Guidelines for management of asthma in adults: II. Acute severe asthma. *BMJ* 1990;**301**: 797-800.
14 Johnson A, Nunn A, Somner A, Stableforth D, Stewart C. Circumstances of death from asthma. *BMJ* 1984;**288**:1870-2.
15 Blainey D, Lomas D, Beale A, Partridge M. The cost of acute asthma—how much is preventable? *Health Trends* 1991;**22**:151-3.
16 Hill RA, Standen PJ, Tattersfield AE. Asthma, wheezing and school absence in primary schools. *Arch Dis Child* 1989;**64**:246-51.
17 Sears MR, Taylor DR, Print CG, Lake DC, Quinquing Li, Flannery EM, *et al*. Regular inhaled β agonist treatment in bronchial asthma. *Lancet* 1990;**336**: 1391-6.
18 Ali NJ, Capewell S, Ward MJ. Bone turnover during high dose inhaled corticosteroid treatment. *Thorax* 1991;**46**:160-4.
19 Wolthers OD, Pedersen S. Growth of asthmatic children during treatment with budesonide: a double blind trial. *BMJ* 1991;**303**:163-5.
20 Hilton S, Sibbald S, Anderson HR, Freeling P. Controlled evaluation of the effects of patient education on asthma morbidity in general practice. *Lancet* 1986;i:26-9.
21 Beasley R, Cushley M, Holgate ST. A self-management plan in the treatment of adult asthma. *Thorax* 1989;**44**:200-4.
22 Charlton I, Charlton G, Bloomfield J, Mullee MA. Evaluation of peak flow and symptoms only self-management plans for control of asthma in general practice. *BMJ* 1990;**301**:1355-9.
23 Bucknall CE, Robertson C, Moran F, Stevenson RD. Differences in hospital asthma management. *Lancet* 1988;i:748-50.
24 Bucknall CE, Robertson C, Moran F, Stevenson RD. Management of asthma in hospital: a prospective audit. *BMJ* 1988;**296**:1637-9.
25 Rees PJ. β_2 agonists and asthma. *BMJ* 1991;**302**:1166-7.
26 Maiman LA, Green LW, Gibson G, MacKenzie EJ. Education for self-treatment by adult asthmatics. *JAMA* 1979;**241**:1919-22.
27 Mayo PH, Richman J, Harris HW. Results of a program to reduce admissions for adult asthma. *Ann Intern Med* 1990;**112**:864-71.

HIV and AIDS

ANNE M JOHNSON

The Health of the Nation described HIV and AIDS as "the greatest new threat to public health this century."[1] Paradoxically, this major area of concern missed the status of a key area on the basis that insufficient prevalence data are currently available to set targets. This is a serious omission for an epidemic which will be most effectively contained by action taken early in its course.

In the emerging culture of management by objectives, managers will increasingly focus on achieving targets set nationally as well as locally through purchaser-provider contracts. The logical outcome is that areas in which targets have not been set will receive both insufficient effort and insufficient resources. Can we therefore afford not to set targets for a pandemic whose aetiology is well understood and for which a clear objective of improvement in safe sexual and injecting drug using behaviours can be set, even if realistic targets for the incidence of disease cannot? This immediately raises a well worn criticism of target setting; that priority is given to only those problems which are measurable.[2] Damage limitation for AIDS and HIV requires early behavioural intervention, and target setting therefore cannot depend solely on the results of unlinked anonymous surveillance of serostatus, which may require data for several further years before clear trends emerge.[3] This leads to a discussion of what constitutes a target.

In *The Health of the Nation* the targets are a mixture of measures of outcome (quantifiable measures of disease incidence and behavioural risk factors) and process measurements (concerned only with health service provision and policy). By contrast, the United States national health objectives, which were produced 10 years before the British strategy, took a broader perspective, identifying objectives in five

---

Government's view on setting targets

An essential first step is to improve understanding of the prevalence of HIV. This knowledge will assist service planning and targeting of public information campaigns. At present the information is insufficient to allow targets to be set for limiting the spread of HIV. The Medical Research Council, funded by the Department of Health, began anonymised surveys of sero-status in January 1990. As these studies become more general-ised their results should enable more accurate predictors of the state and geographic distribution of the epidemic.

---

areas: improving health status; reduced risk factors, increased public and professional awareness; improved services and protection; and improved surveillance and evaluation systems.[4-7] For HIV and AIDS the government considers only measures of health status, concluding that without better estimates of the current magnitude of the epidemic targets cannot be set (box). The Faculty of Public Health Medicine's recent document *UK Levels of Health* and the American report *Healthy people 2000* are not so reluctant and identify sexually transmitted diseases and HIV as priorities and set targets for them.[27] My discussion therefore draws extensively on these documents.

HIV and AIDS as a key area

There is no doubt that HIV and AIDS is a major cause for concern with great potential for future harm. The World Health Organisation estimates that worldwide the total number of people infected with HIV will increase from 9 million to over 15·5 million over the next four years. By 1995, a further half million infected people are expected to be added to the 1·5 million infected in the Western World since the start of the epidemic over 10 years ago. (J Chin, seventh international conference on AIDS, Florence, 1991). The incidence of AIDS is projected to increase and remain high through the 1990s in the developed world, with an increasing proportion of heterosexually acquired infections; the developing world, will also show a consider-able increase in incidence (J Chin, 1991; Public Health Laboratory Service, unpublished data).[8] By 1989, HIV had become the second leading cause of death in America among men aged 25-44 and the eighth leading cause in the same age group of women.[9] In England and Wales the lack of fall in death rates in men aged 15-44 can in part be attributed to HIV related deaths.[10]

Targets for HIV and AIDS have floundered largely on the problems of assessing the rate of spread of HIV in Britain. This is a result of both limited epidemiological data and lack of baseline population estimates of risk behaviour necessary to define the size of behaviour change required to control the epidemic. However, recent results of the unlinked anonymous HIV prevalence studies indicate continued high prevalence and incidence of HIV infection in homosexual men attending genitourinary medicine clinics and increasing rates of infection among women attending antenatal clinics in the Thames regions.[3 11] These, with projections of the future epidemic, provide baseline data from which targets can be set.[3]

Is it rational to single out HIV and AIDS as a key area? It is estimated worldwide that 70-80% of HIV infections are acquired through sexual intercourse and 5-10% through injecting drug use (J Chin, 1991). Similar proportions are reported among patients known to be infected with HIV in the United Kingdom. (Public Health Laboratory Service AIDS Centre *et al* unpublished surveillance table No 11, 1991). HIV is now established as another viral sexually transmitted disease, and its control cannot be separated from that of other sexually acquired infections. More pragmatically, targets might be set for more easily measurable diseases that share the same risk factors, including other sexually transmitted diseases and hepatitis B, as well as for risk reduction, education, and service provision and monitoring.

Much of the management and prevention of sexually transmitted disease in Britain occurs within the network of open access genitourinary medicine clinics, with more than 500 000 attendances annually.[12] The Monks report highlighted the poor state of, and lack of investment in, the service,[13] hardly the environment to provide the health service's mainstay against a major epidemic.

Targets for HIV infection must therefore include service targets within the NHS. But intersectoral and international collaboration is also needed to set targets for statutory and voluntary education services, prison services, travel services, drug services, and overseas development organisations, to name but a few. As HIV emerges as an important problem for the poorest countries and becomes associated with urban deprivation in the West issues of equity, conspicuously absent from discussions in the consultative document, must be addressed.

Setting targets

Improved health

The difficulties of setting precise targets for the incidence of HIV infection reflect the particular characteristics of the disease. The incidence of AIDS reflects infection occurring eight to 10 years earlier, and HIV seroconversion is often asymptomatic and undiagnosed. Targets can be set for reducing the incidence of sexually transmitted diseases, which are more easily measured and less susceptible to changes in service use. For example, reduced incidence of gonorrhoea has been shown to be a useful marker of the adoption of safer sexual practices in homosexual men.[14]

The Faculty of Public Health Medicine has set targets for the incidence of sexually transmitted disease and HIV prevalence, and these provide a basis for discussion.[2] Though national targets may be set, local health authorities may need to set local targets because of the wide geographic variation in the incidences of sexually transmitted disease and HIV.[12]

HIV prevalence

The table summarises the targets for HIV prevalence in the year 2000 set by the Faculty of Public Health Medicine. Targets for homosexual men based on high but stable prevalence may not be sufficiently challenging. As the epidemic matures, there is a substantial annual death rate from HIV infection, and maintaining a constant prevalence may imply a considerable number of newly

Summary of HIV prevalence targets proposed by the Faculty of Public Health Medicine for the year 2000

	Prevalence/1000 population	
	Baseline	Year 2000 target
Male homosexuals attending genitourinary medicine clinics:		
London	200	200
Outside London	50	50
Heterosexuals attending genitourinary medicine clinics (non-injecting drug users):		
London	7	10
Outside London	3	5
Injecting drug users attending services:		
London	20	20
Outside London	10	10

infected people "replacing" those who have died. (T A Kellogg *et al*, seventh international conference on AIDS, Florence, 1991).

Injecting drug users currently have relatively low rates of infection in England and attaining a stable prevalence target will require sustained prevention and treatment efforts for drug users both in and outside treatment for addiction.

Sexually transmitted diseases

The targets for sexually transmitted disease in the year 2000 proposed by the faculty for the population aged 15-64 years may also be useful markers for reduction of risk behaviour for HIV infection. Targets include reducing the incidence of gonorrhoea to no more than 30 cases per 100 000, of chlamydia trachomatis to no more than 75 cases per 100 000, and of infectious syphilis to no more than three per 1 000 000.[2]

Experience in America indicates greater success in achieving targets for gonorrhoea than for syphilis.[15] The faculty's targets are set against rates which are already falling in response to the HIV epidemic, and care must be taken in "plucking figures out of the air" through extrapolation of trends without considering the magnitude of risk reduction necessary to achieve targets.

Age specific targets should also be considered as the highest rates of sexually transmitted diseases are found in the youngest adult age groups, in whom rates of partner change are highest and the age at first intercourse is falling.[16 17]

Reducing risk factors

Measurement of reductions in risk factors for HIV and AIDS is barely addressed by the green paper. Setting targets for reducing risk factors is made difficult by the absence of baseline data on sexual behaviour in the general population, a research topic in which public funding has met with some resistance.[17] Estimates of sexual behaviour will become available from the national survey of sexual attitudes and lifestyles as well as from surveys of knowledge, attitudes, and behaviour undertaken by the Health Education Authority.[18]

These data could be used to set targets for risk reduction, but a strategy for longer term monitoring of risk behaviour is required. Targets worthy of discussion, proposed in the American objectives, include reducing the proportion of under 16 year olds who have had sexual intercourse and increasing the sexually active proportion of unmarried people who used a condom at last sexual intercourse.[7]

Targets for reducing the prevalence of injecting drug use are hampered by the absence of national prevalence data. Monitoring data are becoming available from the national needle exchange programme, and targets could be set both for the proportion of injecting drug users still reporting syringe sharing as well as for safe sex practices. (M C Donoghoe *et al*, seventh international conference on AIDS, Florence, 1991.)

Increased public and professional awareness

Despite recognition of the importance of education in HIV prevention the government set no educational targets. The Faculty of Public Health Medicine proposed "that by the year 2000, all middle and secondary schools should, as part of a wider programme of health promotion, provide education on safer sex behaviours, and on sexually transmitted diseases, including HIV infection and the services available for treatment."[2] This target could usefully be extended to colleges, universities, and other places of higher education and will require close collaboration between the Department of Education and Science and the Health Education Authority.

Training health care workers

The Monks report highlighted the lack of formal training for health advisers in genitourinary medicine clinics.[13] A target might be that by the year 2000 all health advisers should undergo a certificated course, endorsed by the Department of Health, providing appropriate training in the management, counselling, and prevention of HIV infection and sexually transmitted diseases. Educational targets should be extended to other health care staff, particularly those working in primary care, family planning, and genitourinary medicine. Greater consideration should be given to the curriculum for sexual health for medical students, student nurses, and those undergoing higher medical training.

Improved services

An important step towards improved services for prevention of HIV infection and sexually transmitted disease would be the implementation of the Monks report, which set out five priority recommendations and 31 additional recommendations. This document could be used as the basis for standard setting in genitourinary medicine. As a first target, genitourinary medicine services should be provided in every district and additional resources allocated to them by 1995. While local implementation remains the responsibility of regional and district health authorities, monitoring of national progress towards the Monks targets would be most appropriately coordinated by the Department of Health. Monks largely addressed process targets, and the development of measures of outcome, patient satisfaction, and effectiveness needs greater attention.

Services for injecting drug users and policies for treatment need reviewing in the light of the HIV epidemic, and targets might be set for increasing the proportion of drug users receiving treatment for addiction.[7]

Surveillance and evaluation

Progress towards targets requires commitment from management, collaboration between sectors, cost effective resource allocation, and investment in surveillance and evaluation.

Continued anonymous studies of HIV prevalence will be needed to assess progress towards health targets, but to interpret trends greater understanding is required of the relation between incidence and prevalence. Monitoring progress towards targets for sexually transmitted disease can be achieved only by improving timeliness and completeness of disease statistics from the statutory clinic returns (KC60) collated by the Department of Health (currently available only up to 1988). A target for 1995 might be that national figures should be available within six months of the end of the year of collection.

Progress towards educational and risk reduction targets could be achieved by national surveys of knowledge, attitudes, and behaviour. Although the problems of obtaining valid and reliable self reported data on sexual behaviour are recognised, considerable progress has recently been made in question design and assessment of reporting accuracy.[17 19] Adding key questions on sexual behaviour (particularly age at first intercourse, number of sex partners, and condom use) to the national health survey programme discussed in *The Health of the Nation* would be a means of measuring risk reduction. This approach has already been used in America by adding questions to a general social survey and has achieved high acceptance rates.[19] Setting targets for reducing the prevalence of injecting drug use remains impossible unless a national system for monitoring indicators of drug use is established, though needle exchange programmes will provide data on risk reduction.

Measuring service targets, process, and outcome also needs attention. Statutory district annual reports on cases of HIV infection and AIDS and services, produced to comply with the AIDS Control Act, might permit monitoring of targets for genitourinary medicine services. Further research is urgently needed into the content and effectiveness of HIV counselling. Data are not collected routinely on the activity of health advisers and data on tracing of contacts of patients with sexually transmitted diseases have been dropped from routine Department of Health returns. As such work is one of the mainstays of prevention of sexually transmitted disease further work on activity and outcome measurement is needed, not least on understanding the determinants of risk behaviour and risk reduction.

Equity and collaboration

A strategy for controlling the spread of HIV must consider global responses to the pandemic. Sexually transmitted diseases have never been respecters of international borders (despite the attempts of some governments to make them so). Any increased spread in Britain will be reflected worldwide and vice versa. Targets for controlling HIV cannot therefore be divorced from questions of international collaboration to support the countries of sub Saharan Africa, South and South East Asia, and Latin America economically and in control programmes for HIV and sexually transmitted disease. Equity must be addressed nationally and internationally. In America attention has recently been drawn to the association between social deprivation in the inner cities, particularly among ethnic minorities, and spread of HIV.[20] It is those who are most socially disadvantaged who may be increasingly affected by the epidemic through drug use, unsafe sex, and economic reliance on the sex industry. Social, educational, and fiscal measures directed towards these inequalities are therefore an integral part of the control of HIV infection.

In conclusion, targets can be set for control of HIV and AIDS, particularly when the definition of a target is not limited to measuring health status. Statutory and voluntary agencies across a spectrum of disciplines need to define a strategy for preventing the spread of HIV infection. They should not allow HIV to be forgotten in setting the future foundations of the health of the nation.

1 Secretary of State for Health. *The Health of the Nation*. London: HMSO, 1991.
2 The Faculty of Public Health Medicine of the Royal College of Physicians. *UK levels of health. First report*. London: FPHM, 1991.
3 Public Health Laboratory Service AIDS Centre and Viral Research Laboratory. Academic Department of Genitourinary Medicine, University College and Middlesex School of

Medicine, and collaborators. The unlinked anonymous HIV prevalence monitoring programme in England and Wales: preliminary results. *Communicable Disease Report* 1991; No 1:R69-76.

4 Public Health Service. *Healthy people: the Surgeon General's report on health promotion and disease prevention.* Washington, DC: Department of Health, Education and Welfare, Public Health Service, 1979. (DHEW publication (PHS) 79-55071.)

5 Public Health Service. *Promoting health/preventing diseases: objectives for the Nation.* Washington, DC: Department of Health and Human Services, Public Health Service, 1980.

6 McGinnis JM. Setting nationwide objectives in disease prevention and health promotion: the United States experience. Holland WW, Detels R, Knox G, eds. *Oxford Textbook of Public Health Medicine.* Oxford: Oxford University Press, 1985:385-401.

7 Public Health Service. *Healthy people 2000: national health promotion and disease prevention objectives.* Washington, DC: Department of Health and Human Services, Public Health Service, 1990. (DHHS publication no (PHS) 90-50212.)

8 Brookmeyer R. Reconstruction and future trends of the AIDS epidemic in the United States. *Science* 1991;253:37-42.

9 Centers for Disease Control. Mortality attributable to HIV infection/AIDS—United States, 1981-1990. *MMWR* 1990;40:41-5.

10 Dunnell K. Deaths amongst 15-44 year olds. *Population Trends* 1991;64:38-43.

11 Ades AE, Parker S, Berry T, Holland FJ, Davison CF, Cubitt D, *et al.* Prevalence of maternal HIV-1 infection in Thames regions: results from anonymous unlinked neonatal testing. *Lancet* 1991;337:1562-5.

12 Department of Health. *New cases seen at NHS genitourinary medicine clinics in England. 1988 annual and December quarter figures. Summary information from form KC60.* London: DoH, 1990.

13 Working Group to Examine Workloads in Genitourinary Medicine Clinics. *Report.* London: Department of Health, 1988. (Chairman A Monks.)

14 Johnson AM, Gill ON. Evidence for recent changes in sexual behaviour in homosexual men in England and Wales. *Philos Trans R Soc Lond [Biol]* 1989;325:115-25.

15 Centers for Disease Control. Progress towards achieving the 1990 objectives for the nation for sexually transmitted diseases. *MMWR* 1990;39:54-7.

16 Johnson AM, Wadsworth J, Elliott P, Prior L, Wallace P, Blowers S, *et al.* A pilot study of sexual behaviour in a random sample of the population of Great Britain. *AIDS* 1989;3: 135-41.

17 Wellings K, Wadsworth J, Field J, Anderson RM, Bradshaw SA. Sexual lifestyles under scrutiny. *Nature* 1990;348:276-8.

18 Health Education Authority. *AIDS strategic monitor: report on the survey period November 1987-December 1988.* London: HEA, 1988.

19 Centers for Disease Control. Number of sex partners and potential risk of sexual exposure to human immunodeficiency virus. *MMWR* 1988;37:565-8.

20 Wodak A, Moss A. HIV infection and injecting drugs users: from epidemiology to public health. *AIDS* 1990;4(suppl 1):S105-9.

Strategy for stroke

MARTIN DENNIS, CHARLES WARLOW

In the consultation document for health in England the government identified stroke as a possible priority for disease prevention and treatment.[1] We will consider how well stroke fulfils the criteria for a key area, what targets should be set, how we might achieve them, and what the problems are likely to be, particularly in monitoring any progress.

Making stroke a priority

The first criterion for a key area is that it should be a major cause of premature death or avoidable ill health either in the population as a whole or among specific groups of people. About 100 000 people each year have a first stroke in England; about 25 000 are less than 65 years old and another 29 000 are aged between 65 and 74.[2] Each year 64 000 deaths are attributed to stroke in England, representing 12% of all deaths.[1] Of these, 5000 deaths occur in those under 65 years and 11 000 in those aged 65-75 (5% and 9% of all deaths in each age category respectively).[1]

Stroke is also one of the commonest causes of severe disability.[3] Furthermore it consumes vast resources. Isard and Forbes estimated that in Scotland in 1988 stroke accounted for about 4·3% of all NHS resources and 5·5% of hospital resources.[4] The costs to patients, their families, and society must be huge but have never been quantified. Also it is a disease which even in Britain particularly affects certain ethnic groups[5] and the socially deprived.[6] Thus stroke is clearly an important avoidable cause of premature death and disability.

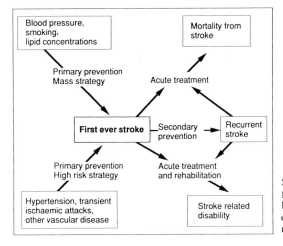

Strategies
for improving health
by reducing incidence
of stroke and associated
mortality and disability

Effective interventions

The government's second criterion is that there should be effective interventions and scope for improvement in health. Certainly over the past 20 years most developed countries have seen a reduction in mortality from stroke (by 2-7% a year[7]), and this may be due to a fall in incidence of stroke,[8] although there is no definite evidence that the incidence is falling in England as the discussion document wrongly asserts.[1] Most of the observed reduction in mortality is unexplained, although the treatment of hypertension may have played some part.[9]

The figure shows the interventions which would reduce the incidence of stroke and associated mortality and disability. Some interventions, for instance primary and secondary prevention, would reduce not just the incidence but also mortality and disability. Others, such as rehabilitation, will reduce only disability.

Primary prevention

Primary prevention can be approached in two ways: the "mass strategy" and the "high risk strategy."[10] The risk factors for stroke are qualitatively if not quantitatively the same as for coronary heart disease, another possible key area, so for practical purposes they should be considered together. In the mass strategy the aim is to reduce the prevalence or shift the distribution of a risk factor across the entire population. A modest 5 mm Hg reduction in mean population diastolic blood pressure, achievable by reducing the mean

93

daily salt intake in the population by 50 mmol/l, might reduce mortality from stroke by 22%.[11] By reducing salt in processed food a reduction in mean salt intake of 100 mmol/l a day could be achieved, which might reduce the incidence of and mortality from stroke by 39%.[11] Further reductions in blood pressure might be derived by reducing the population's alcohol intake and obesity.

We could perhaps further reduce the incidence of stroke, especially in the young, by substantially reducing the prevalence of cigarette smoking, which increases the risk of stroke, by 50%.[12] The role of lipids in stroke is still unclear, but improvement in diet would probably reduce the incidence of ischaemic stroke as well as that of coronary heart disease. The cost and possible adverse effects of such mass strategies are difficult to estimate.

High risk strategies include identifying and treating people with hypertension and other established vascular disease. Treatment of all hypertensive people (>100 mm Hg diastolic pressure) in the population might reduce mortality from stroke by about 15%.[11] The risk of stroke (and other vascular events) in patients who have had transient ischaemic attacks can be reduced not just by modifying their risk factors but by using aspirin, which will reduce the risk of subsequent stroke by about 25%.[13] Carotid endarterectomy would further reduce the risk of stroke in suitable patients.[14] However, only 15% of patients with stroke have had previous transient ischaemic attacks; many of those who have had an attack do not present to a doctor and not all of those who do present are eligible for specific treatment. For example, about 5000 of the 20 000 patients presenting to a doctor in England with transient ischaemic attack each year may be suitable for carotid endarterectomy. The 5000 operations might prevent about 500 first strokes a year, representing a 0·5% reduction in incidence of first stroke. Aspirin, which is more widely applicable, may reduce the overall incidence of stroke by 1-2%, although even this reduction is an order of magnitude lower than that which could be achieved using the mass strategies described above. Another problem with the high risk strategy is that to be effective it would require a large scale screening or case finding programme and then even greater effort to provide treatment and follow up.[15]

Secondary prevention

After a first stroke the risk of recurrence is about 13% in the first year and about 5% in each year thereafter. The modification of vascular risk factors, treatment with aspirin, and carotid endarterectomy all have a role in secondary prevention and would reduce the overall incidence of stroke and associated mortality and disability.

Acute treatment

Treatments to reduce brain injury after acute stroke have great potential for reducing mortality and disability but none has yet been shown to be effective. Randomised trials of acute treatment have been too small to show clinically worthwhile effects of treatment, and efforts to carry out large trials are hampered by lack of resources for clinical research, interest, and acute stroke units. Simple inexpensive treatments such as aspirin, which could be given to most patients with acute stroke even if found to be only moderately effective, may yield important overall effects. For example, if 90% of all patients with acute stroke were given a drug that reduces the risk of death and disability by only 20% about 15 000 patients would be saved from death or disability in England each year.

Rehabilitation

Once the patient has had a stroke we have little to offer apart from effective rehabilitation. But stroke services in Britain are poorly organised,[16] and many patients fail to achieve their maximum potential for recovery. Although few randomised trials of stroke rehabilitation have been conducted, there is some evidence that organised stroke units can achieve more rapid functional improvement.[17] A lot of our efforts in rehabilitation are unfocused; without further research to give us precise estimates of the relative effectiveness of different aspects of rehabilitation it is impossible to predict the overall benefit that better organised rehabilitation could have on disability and handicap.

Setting and monitoring targets

The third criterion is that it should be possible to set objectives and targets in the chosen topic and to monitor progress towards their achievement through indicators. The government's targets for reducing mortality by 30% in people aged under 65 and 25% in those aged 65-74 by the year 2000 are ambitious (box) as the effects of changes in lifestyle will inevitably be delayed. Nevertheless, because treating blood pressure has an effect on risk of stroke within two to three years the targets are probably reasonable.[18] They might be reached by reducing the incidence of stroke by similar amounts.

Government's possible targets for stroke

Reduction in premature death
- Between 1988 and 2000 achieve a 30% reduction in mortality from stroke in people aged less than 65
- Reduce mortality from stroke by 25% in people aged 65-74 over the same period

Other targets
Views on other targets are welcomed. Possibilities include:
- Reducing the incidence of stroke
- Local or national screening for and treatment of hypertension
- Proportion of people surviving stroke able to live outside institutional care after given period

---

Difficulties arise in developing reliable methods to monitor progress towards these goals. This problem might be the main reason for not identifying stroke as a key area, although it must be an equal or even greater problem in other suggested key areas.

Mortality from stroke is the easiest target to assess or monitor but it depends on the accuracy of death certification, which is especially poor in elderly people.[19] If monitoring of mortality was restricted to those less than 70 years old it would be more accurate and might allow interpretation of geographic and secular trends. We could then concentrate on reducing death rates in areas with the highest rates down to those in areas with the lowest rates, possibly by focusing on regional differences in diet, smoking habits, and social deprivation. Unless there are changes in fashion in death certification, the mortality from stroke is likely to be a fairly reliable indicator of change. Such a change may also reflect changes in incidence, although if the case fatality rate should alter—for example, because of the introduction of an effective acute treatment—then this may no longer be so.

Ideally the incidence of first and recurrent strokes should be monitored as this would give a direct measure of success in primary and secondary prevention. Measuring the incidence of stroke is tiresome but not difficult,[2] but it could not be achieved nationally unless stroke was a notifiable disease. Simply counting people admitted to or discharged from hospital with stroke could be misleading as the proportion of patients with stroke admitted to hospital varies greatly in different places[8] and is likely to change over time, especially with the NHS reforms. It would be possible, however, and not very expensive, to set up perhaps 10 studies to monitor stroke incidence in carefully selected and representative parts of the country. The methods would have to be identical and fulfil criteria laid down by Malmgrem *et al*[8] and the study populations large enough to provide reliable data. Ideally they would be combined with studies of other vascular diseases, such as coronary heart disease, to make the best use of resources.

To monitor changes in disability due to stroke would present considerable methodological problems. Direct measures of disability (for example, Barthel score) are not collected widely, and although indirect measures such as place and timing of discharge from hospital are collected, these are dependent on local community facilities (for example, adequate housing, good community care, etc), which also tend to change over time. Also, the most important factor in determining the disability of patients discharged from hospital is not the quality or amount of rehabilitation but the severity of stroke in patients admitted to hospital—that is, case mix. The questions of how and when to measure outcome, how outcome may relate to case mix, how its measurement can be done on a large enough scale to show progress towards a target, and how much its measurement will cost must be investigated in future health services research. An alternative approach would be to repeat the disability survey[3] regularly to determine whether the prevalence of disability caused by stroke is falling, but it is difficult to distinguish reliably between stroke related disability and that resulting from other diseases. Until a satisfactory measure of stroke related disability or handicap is identified it would seem premature to follow this option.

One solution would be to substitute measures of process until satisfactory measures of outcome and case mix have been developed. Process measures would, however, be indirect and possibly distract from the real issue of outcome. Possible measures include the proportions of health districts with an identified person responsible for stroke services,[16] a stroke unit, or a strategy for stroke or the proportion of patients with a recent blood pressure, weight, and smoking history in their general practitioners' records.

Conclusions

Improvements in the nation's health with respect to stroke could be achieved by primary prevention. The greatest effect is likely to be achieved with a mass strategy focusing on salt, alcohol, and fat intake and smoking. These issues go far wider than the Department of Health and the NHS and whether the political will exists to carry through such policies is open to debate. Health education alone may not be effective and would need to be backed up by legislation (for example, food labelling for salt content, ban on tobacco advertising) and financial incentives (taxing tobacco and alcohol). By encouraging effective screening or case finding and treating high risk individuals with interventions that have been properly evaluated in randomised trials, by developing effective treatments for acute stroke, and by improving rehabilitation services extra benefits are possible. Such interventions are, however, no substitute for the mass strategy. Some improvements could be monitored simply but rather unreliably by looking at changes in mortality, but we need to develop practical and inexpensive methods for routine monitoring of the incidence and outcome of stroke.

1 Secretary of State for Health. *The health of the nation*. London: HMSO, 1991. (Cm 1523.)
2 Bamford J, Sandercock P, Dennis M, Warlow C, Jones L, McPherson K, *et al*. A prospective study of acute cerebrovascular disease in the community: the Oxfordshire community stroke project, 1981-86. 1. Methodology, demography and incident cases of first-ever stroke. *J Neurol Neurosurg Psychiatry* 1988;**51**:1373-80.
3 Office of Population Censuses and Surveys. *The prevalence of disability among adults*. London: HMSO, 1988.
4 Isard P, Forbes J. The cost of stroke to the NHS in Scotland. *Cerebrovascular Diseases* (in press).
5 Balarajan R. Ethnic differences in mortality from ischaemic heart disease and cerebrovascular disease in England and Wales. *BMJ* 1991;**302**:560-4.
6 Carstairs V, Morris R. Deprivation and health in Scotland. *Health Bull (Edinb)* 1990;**48**:162-75.
7 Bonita R, Stewart A, Beaglehole R. International trends in stroke mortality: 1970-1985. *Stroke* 1990;**21**:989-92.
8 Malmgren R, Warlow C, Bamford J, Sandercock P. Geographical and secular trends in stroke incidence. *Lancet* 1987;ii:1196-200.
9 Bonita R, Beaglehole R. Does treatment of hypertension explain the decline in mortality from stroke? *BMJ* 1986;**292**:191-2.
10 Rose G. Strategy of prevention: lessons from cardiovascular disease. *BMJ* 1981;**282**:1847-51.
11 Law M, Frost C, Wald N. By how much does dietary salt reduction lower blood pressure. III. Analysis of data from trials of salt reduction. *BMJ* 1991;**302**:819-24.
12 Shinton R, Beevers G. Meta-analysis of relation between cigarette smoking and stroke. *BMJ* 1989;**298**:789-94.
13 Antiplatelet Trialists Collaboration. Secondary prevention of vascular disease by prolonged antiplatelet treatment. *BMJ* 1988;**296**:320-31.
14 European Carotid Surgery Trialists' Collaborative Group. MRC European Carotid Surgery trial: interim results for symptomatic patients with severe (70-99%) or with mild (0·29%) carotid stenosis. *Lancet* 1991;**337**:1235-43.
15 Imperial Cancer Research Fund OXCHECK Study Group. Prevalence of risk factors for heart disease in OXCHECK trial: implications for screening in primary care. *BMJ* 1991;**302**:1057-60.

16 King's Fund Consensus Conference. Treatment of stroke. *BMJ* 1988;**297**: 1268.

17 Garraway WM, Akhtar A, Prescott R, Hockey L. Management of acute stroke in the elderly: preliminary results of a controlled trial. *BMJ* 1980;**280**: 1040-3.

18 Collins R, Peto R, MacMahon S, Herbert P, Fiebach N, Eberlein K, *et al*. Blood pressure, stroke, and coronary heart disease. 2. Short-term reductions in blood pressure: overview of randomised drug trials in their epidemiological context. *Lancet* 1990;**335**:827-38.

19 Cameron HM, McGoogan E. A prospective study of 1152 hospital autopsies. 1. Inaccuracies in death certification. *J Pathol* 1981;**133**:273-83.

Communicable diseases other than AIDS

NORMAN D NOAH

Should communicable diseases be a key area?

Superficially, the case against communicable diseases other than AIDS and HIV infection being a key area of great concern in the United Kingdom for targeting action is quite strong. Most infectious diseases are mild; even influenza A virus, the last great organism until HIV capable of causing a pandemic, has been fairly quiescent for 15 or so years; and mass immunisation and sanitation have kept many of the former scourges in check. In *The Health of the Nation*, however, communicable diseases are chosen as a key area but not because they are considered to cause substantial mortality or substantial ill health or to have scope for improvement. Instead, they are included in the group "where there is great potential for harm."[1] This implies either that they are not serious at present but may become so or that many of the most serious conditions are under control at present but may revert if control is relaxed. This underestimates the contribution of communicable disease to general ill health.

The first criterion for the choice of a key area is that the disease should be a major cause of premature death or avoidable ill health in the general population or in specific groups of people. With the possible exception of influenza—and the length of time since a major epidemic leaves no room for complacency—communicable diseases are not major causes of premature death. Nevertheless, by their very diversity and frequency they are certainly major causes of ill health; many of them are avoidable, at least in the sense that we know what causes them and how they are transmitted. The sexually transmitted diseases not only cause an acute self limiting illness but also give rise to sequelae, including pelvic inflammatory disease, ectopic pregnancy, infertility, and carcinoma (of the penis, cervix, and anus), as well as congenital abnormalities and neonatal illness. Some communicable diseases recur or become chronic, and the lesions in sexually transmitted disease may facilitate the transmission of HIV and probably hepatitis B. Infectious diarrhoea and respiratory and urinary tract infections are further examples of major causes of ill health, though how much is avoidable is debatable and difficult to estimate.

The second criterion for a key area is that effective intervention is possible. Apart from sanitation and immunisation, what other effective interventions are there against communicable disease? High up on this list I would place effective surveillance and control of outbreaks: the early recognition of outbreaks through effective surveillance is undoubtedly an important form of secondary prevention. Antibiotics are useful in preventing the sequelae of and death from many communicable diseases, but they are generally disappointing in preventing the disease and may even induce complacency.

Targets for communicable disease

The third criterion for a key area is the ability to set objectives and targets and to monitor progress. Targets can be set in communicable disease, but apart from detailing the obvious one of immunisation rates *The Health of the Nation* is curiously negative about possible targets (box). Sexually transmitted diseases are mentioned briefly in a paragraph appended to the section on HIV and AIDS and no targets are set. Targets for hospital acquired infection "could be set on the basis of what can be achieved through good practice," and for microbiological food poisoning we need to wait for the results of studies by the Department of Health and "analysis of activities

---

Possible targets for communicable diseases

- 95% rates of immunisation against diphtheria, tetanus, polio, measles, mumps, rubella, and whooping cough
- 90% reduction on 1989 values of notifications of measles by 1995
- Audit of hospital acquired infections in individual units to set realistic targets for reduction

---

of enforcement officers" because "there is currently no sound basis for determining targets for reductions in incidence of foodborne diseases."[1]

Are these realistic approaches to communicable disease targets? If not, what should the targets be? The Faculty of Public Health Medicine in its report *UK Levels of Health*, which appeared at the same time as *The Health of the Nation*, is less conservative in its approach,[2] and I will consider some of its recommendations with those of the government.

Immunisation—Targets are straightforward when a disease has a vaccine. Most such diseases have so low an incidence that they are no longer a public health problem (the definition of containment), and they may quite reasonably be classified as "areas where there is great potential for harm." For all of these diseases except one the target is the rate of immunisation rather than the prevalence of the disease. The exception is measles, for which the target is to reduce the notification rate to 10% of its 1989 rate—that is, less than 3000 cases a year in England and Wales by 1995. This sets a further challenge to health authorities, most of which have already achieved the WHO target of a 90% reduction in measles from the rates recorded before immunisation began in 1968. *UK Levels of Health* sets targets for measles of 5000 cases a year by 1995 (including Scotland) and 1000 by the year 2000. It sets even lower targets for pertussis, mumps, and rubella and suggests that there should be no cases of the congenital rubella syndrome (without mention of abortions for rubella), polio, or diphtheria by the year 2000.[2]

Sexually transmitted diseases—*The Health of the Nation* acknowledges sexually transmitted diseases to be important and disabling but no targets are discussed or set. Although there are no absolute data on incidences, returns from clinics to the Department of Health are reasonable indicators of trends. *UK Levels of Health* does set targets but does not state how they are arrived at (table).[2]

Hospital acquired infection—It is undoubtedly difficult to set targets for hospital acquired infection. As different hospitals may vary in their infection rates national standards are not warranted. A useful approach, however, could be for each hospital to establish a hospital infection surveillance and control structure,[3] which is in itself a target; determine its infection rate in different categories (wound infections, urinary tract infections, etc); and then set its own targets.

Foodborne illness—Targets are also difficult to set for foodborne illness. Unlike those for sexually transmitted diseases, routine

Rates in 1988, based on clinic returns to Department of Health, and target rates for year 2000 of sexually transmitted diseases (per 100 000 population aged 15-64)[2]

Disease	1988	2000
Gonorrhoea	64·0	30·0
Syphilis	15	3
Congenital syphilis	3	0
Chlamydia trachomatis infection	120	75
Genital herpes	56·2	40·0

statistics for food poisoning are not detailed enough. Nevertheless, as for hospital acquired infection, targets could be set on good practices; it is surprising that the recommendations, of which there were more than 100, of the Committee on the Microbiological Safety of Food are not mentioned.[4] Better knowledge of simple hygiene measures, such as keeping cooked food either very hot or very cold and preventing cross contamination from raw to cooked food among both catering staff and household cooks would go a long way towards reducing microbiological food hazards. Good manufacturing practice in industry, including the endorsement of the hazard analysis and critical control point system (HACCP) used by most food manufacturers, could also be a target.

Strategy

The strategy chosen in *The Health of the Nation* to achieve the targets for communicable disease include immunisation, effective surveillance and control of outbreaks, early diagnosis, and health education for immunisation. Only immunisation is developed any further and control of outbreaks is directed at the human rather than the environmental source of outbreaks. Early diagnosis is to allow appropriate treatment and is presumably targeted at bacterial meningitis. Late diagnosis of meningitis is reported from time to time, but it is probably not a common problem. Health education for immunisation should be targeted at health care workers as much as at the public.

Sexually transmitted diseases—In *The Health of the Nation* "health education and other preventive activities are the key" to reducing sexually transmitted diseases. The opportunity could perhaps be seized to be more specific about these worrying diseases that are difficult to control. Teaching on safe sexual practices and family

103

planning in all middle and secondary schools should be part of a general programme of health education aimed at children. *UK Levels of Health* also adds effective contact tracing and appropriate training for all physicians in counselling on the prevention of sexually transmitted diseases.[2]

Hospital acquired infection is undoubtedly an important area for control (as recognised in *The Health of the Nation* but not in *UK Levels of Health*), but targets and strategy for control are least well developed. As I mentioned earlier possible effective strategy for control includes an effective hospital infection surveillance and control structure in all hospitals, with a responsible hospital infection control nurse or officer.[3]

Food poisoning—A detailed list of reduced risk factors in food poisoning is included in *UK Levels of Health*, but a strategy for the control of food poisoning needs careful thought. It should nevertheless be possible. As recommended by the Richmond committee,[4] two government committees have been established and will need to be consulted.

Local authorities—The responsibilities of several central government departments are detailed in chapter 4 of *The Health of the Nation*. Local authorities, particularly environmental health departments, are mentioned only briefly. Their role in the strategy for control of communicable diseases, especially food poisoning, needs to be acknowledged more positively.

Problems in achieving targets

Any additional resources to achieve the targets in *The Health of the Nation* will probably not be available. For example, the phrase "Teaching on safe sexual practices and family planning in all middle and secondary schools" picked almost at random from the strategy section conceals an enormous amount of work, continuous motivation, organisation, and funding.

To achieve targets good information is needed, and obtaining good information is likely to be the biggest problem. Moreover, the surveillance needs for each key area are different: some have yet to be developed and others improved. To achieve immunisation targets requires not only efficient computers but also staff to key in the data and a rapid information retrieval system. In additon, the special payments to general practitioners to achieve the targets in their practices may have a negative effect in that general practitioners who believe that they cannot achieve the minimum level of 70% for payment may not try to increase a low level of uptake or halt a declining uptake.

Omissions

Here is a personal selection of omissions from *The Health of the Nation*. Though effective sanitation is taken for granted, the faecal-oral cycle is still completed with unacceptable regularity. Scares about the supply of tap water occur from time to time. Studies on the safety of British bathing beaches are in progress, but the high risk of gastroenteritis after eating raw oysters already provides clear evidence of sewage pollution of the sea.[5]

More than 5000 cases of tuberculosis are notified in England and Wales each and every year. This disease, although preventable, is therefore still a problem in many districts, and an effective strategy to reduce its incidence is needed. Legionnaires' disease is also preventable: guidelines are available for hygienic maintenance of hot water systems and cooling towers. There is evidence that even sporadic cases of legionnaires' disease are associated with cooling towers,[6] and the BBC and Stafford outbreaks showed clearly how vulnerable large numbers of people may be in densely populated areas.[7][8] Finally, it seems absurd that we are trying to develop complex targets for health while the sale of unpasteurised milk, if only in England and Wales, is still permitted.

1 Secretary of State for Health. *The Health of the Nation*. London: HMSO, 1991.
2 Faculty of Public Health Medicine of the Royal College of Physicians. *UK levels of health. First report*. London: Faculty of Public Health Medicine 1991. (Chairman: Professor W W Holland.)
3 Department of Health and Social Security. *Hospital infection control: guidance on the control of infection in hospitals prepared by the joint DHSS/PHLS Hospital Infection Working Group*. London: DHSS, 1988. (Chairman: Professor E M Cooke.)
4 Committee on the Microbiological Safety of Food. *The microbiological safety of food*. London: HMSO, 1990. (Chairman: Sir Mark Richmond.)
5 Heller D, Gill ON, Raynham E, Kirkland T, Zadick PM, Stanwell-Smith R. An outbreak of gastrointestinal illness associated with consumption of raw depurated oysters. *BMJ* 1986;**292**: 1726-7.
6 Bhopal RS, Fallon RJ, Buist EC, Black RJ, Urquhart JD. Proximity of the home to a cooling tower and risk of non-outbreak legionnaires' disease. *BMJ* 1991;**302**:378-83.
7 Westminster Action Committee. *Broadcasting House legionnaires' disease: report of the Westminster Action Committee convened to co-ordinate the investigation and control of the outbreak of legionnaires' disease associated with Portland Place, London W1, in April/May 1988*. London: City of Westminster, 1988. (Chairman: Dr D Cunningham.)
8 O'Mahony MC, Stanwell-Smith RE, Tillett HE, Harper D, Hutchison JGP, Farrell ID, *et al.* The Stafford outbreak of legionnaires' disease. *Epidemiol Infect* 1990;**104**:361-80.

Coronary heart disease

HUGH TUNSTALL-PEDOE

The case for coronary heart disease being a key area?

The Secretary of State for Health's consultative document *The Health of the Nation* has appropriately listed coronary heart disease first among 16 suggested key areas.[1] It is difficult to envisage a health strategy for England without including coronary heart disease at the top. The document's primary criteria for designating key areas are that they are major causes of premature death, of avoidable ill health, and of economic cost to the NHS and the community. Several diseases rank highly for one criterion alone, but coronary heart disease, the major contributor to cardiovascular disease, is at or near the top in all three. It is the leading cause of death in both sexes and is estimated to cost annually £500m in treatment and £1800m in lost production, besides having accounted for 11·6% of sick leave, in the mid-1980s.[2]

Other criteria are that the disease should be one in which effective interventions are possible, objectives and targets can be set, and progress can be monitored by means of indicators. Again, coronary heart disease is the chronic disease on which the greatest volume of research has been done: into causation and risk factors (prevention or risk reduction), as well as into monitoring trends in risk factors and the progression of the disease in cohort studies, randomised groups, and geographically defined populations.

A final criterion, for those concerned with reducing inequality, is that mortality from coronary heart disease shows large differences between nations (England scores badly), between English regions and districts (bad for the north and west and the traditional smoke stack areas), between different occupational social classes (bad for manual workers), between ethnic groups (bad for south Asians), and between

106

the sexes (men die earlier and women suffer disproportionate bereavement thereby). Effective coronary prevention has great potential for reducing some of these differences.

What is the case against?

Many of the arguments against making coronary heart disease a key area for a national strategy for health would be those against having such a strategy at all and will not be discussed specifically. Over the past 10 years the case for England not joining other nations in designating coronary heart disease as a key target for a national strategy has been weakened by what has happened elsewhere. Other countries have got their act together and achieved a national consensus for action through collaboration among government agencies, professional bodies, and voluntary organisations. And mortality has fallen even faster. Britain seems to have been acting as the control for other English speaking nations. Although Britain has produced some outstanding researchers and teachers in cardiovascular epidemiology and prevention, there has been national inertia on prevention. This has been justified by the mistaken argument that as long as one or more academics argue against the prevalent hypotheses, that there are two sides to the argument, the experts therefore disagree and it is safer, wiser, and cheaper to do nothing. The decline in coronary heart disease mortality in Britain has been delayed.

The association between these phenomena for Britain versus several European and English speaking countries is undoubted; the causal relation is not entirely straightforward. A declining mortality and the changing lifestyles and social attitudes against which it is occurring are far more conducive to a prevention programme than one in which mortality is static or rising. The comparative success of the Belgian versus the United Kingdom heart disease prevention project in the early 1970s is usually ascribed to more intensive intervention in the Belgian study and is correlated with the greater overall change in risk factors.[3] In fact, the greatest study induced change in self reported cigarette smoking occurred in factories in Britain, where stopping smoking was well established. By contrast, there was virtually no impact of dietary counselling on blood cholesterol concentration in the British factories. It had no support or echoes in the men's previous knowledge or everyday experience. Perhaps its time had not yet come.

Coronary prevention therefore faces a paradox. When the disease is

107

still rising or at its peak the task may be difficult and not widely accepted. When mortality and risk factor levels are declining already the purist could (and some do) argue that no purpose is served by interfering further. A cynic could claim that the guaranteed success of a prevention programme makes it politically desirable. A realist would claim that accelerating and generalising a beneficial trend may be the most cost effective point for concerted action. It may also be true that the general population is prepared to take greater efforts to avoid a disease that is seen to be declining and associated with life's losers than when it is claimed to be the price of a modern lifestyle and executive success.

Another argument used against making coronary heart disease a specific target is that a health strategy should concentrate on health rather than specific diseases. Though it is true that diseases cannot be considered in isolation, the health argument at worst can become metaphysical and untestable. Unless major causes of mortality and morbidity are improved by a health strategy it cannot be considered to be successful. Coronary heart disease should be an identified target but integrated, as in this document, with other diseases, and with lifestyles and risk factors of general relevance.

What should the targets be?

The consultative document has suggested that the primary target for coronary heart disease should be a 30% reduction nationally in the numbers of deaths in people under 65 between 1988 and the year 2000 (box). Elsewhere in the document it is explained that what is meant is the death rate standardised to the World Health Organisation's European standard population.[4] This target is simple and measurable as it depends on routine death certification. It is subject to question, firstly, on the size of the target and, secondly, in that it addresses mortality alone and not morbidity or economic cost.

Mortality from coronary heart disease is a moving target—the baseline is not level, and therefore the target mortality is not 30% lower than it would have been without the intervention. The tables show data on England and Wales analysed from a printout provided by WHO. Tables I and II show mortality from coronary heart disease (ICD code 410-414) in men and women by five year age groups from the age of 30 to the age of 69. In 1972 rates were on the high point of a plateau, just before a decline; 1989 is the latest available year. The penultimate column in each table (including table III) shows the rates as standardised to the WHO European standard population (weighted 7 for each age group under 55, 6 for those aged 55-59, and 5 for those aged 60-64, and then divided by 46), and the final column shows the all ages rate without any standardisation (reflecting changes in mortality across all age groups and also the increasing proportion of

TABLE I—Mortality from coronary heart disease in England and Wales in men by age group and year. Mortality is expressed as rate per 100 000 and as percentages of rate in 1972

Year	Age group (years)									
	30-34	35-39	40-44	45-49	50-54	55-59	60-64	65-69	30-64*	Total
1972	10·9	36·9	95·1	213·8	365·9	576·5	898·7	1417·6	282·8	366·9
1973	10·9	35·2	93·2	210·1	360·0	574·4	885·2	1390·1	279·1	364·4
	100·0	95·4	98·0	98·3	98·4	99·6	98·5	98·1	98·7	99·3
1974	10·4	33·7	96·4	202·7	368·6	573·7	883·5	1383·2	279·2	367·0
	95·4	91·3	101·0	94·8	100·7	99·5	98·3	97·6	98·7	100·0
1975	11·0	30·6	91·8	201·3	375·0	559·0	882·5	1375·0	276·8	370·7
	100·9	82·9	96·5	94·2	102·5	97·0	98·2	97·0	97·9	101·0
1976	9·0	32·9	85·6	188·5	352·9	576·9	890·8	1360·9	273·9	373·5
	82·6	89·2	90·0	88·2	96·5	100·0	99·1	96·0	96·9	101·8
1977	9·3	31·5	88·3	187·6	355·1	564·7	873·1	1367·5	270·8	373·8
	85·3	85·4	92·9	87·8	97·1	98·0	97·2	96·5	95·8	101·9
1978	8·2	35·8	88·0	189·7	367·3	579·1	920·9	1381·7	280·5	386·3
	75·2	97·0	92·5	88·7	100·4	100·5	102·5	97·5	99·2	105·3
1979	10·0	30·5	80·8	189·1	362·1	581·9	926·1	1339·1	278·9	378·1
	91·7	82·7	85·0	88·5	99·0	100·9	103·1	94·5	98·6	103·1
1980	8·9	29·8	80·3	176·1	347·9	577·2	879·3	1314·6	268·7	373·8
	81·7	80·8	84·4	82·4	95·1	100·1	97·8	92·7	95·1	101·9
1981	10·0	28·7	75·9	170·6	326·8	544·4	837·0	1270·8	255·1	369·4
	91·7	77·8	79·8	79·8	89·3	94·4	93·1	89·6	90·2	100·7
1982	9·0	24·7	71·8	157·3	315·2	535·7	826·5	1269·4	247·4	367·4
	82·6	66·9	75·5	73·6	86·1	92·9	92·0	89·5	87·6	100·1
1983	8·2	25·2	68·2	163·5	303·3	531·0	836·7	1316·9	246·7	370·3
	75·2	68·3	71·7	76·5	82·9	92·1	93·1	92·9	87·2	100·9
1984	7·9	22·1	62·4	150·7	287·0	521·7	829·5	1280·4	238·9	366·8
	72·5	59·9	65·6	70·5	78·4	90·5	92·3	90·3	84·5	100·0
1985	6·3	22·8	63·9	146·6	286·8	499·1	841·5	1252·8	236·7	376·6
	57·8	61·8	67·2	68·6	78·4	86·6	93·6	88·4	83·7	102·6
1986	7·1	24·4	59·4	141·6	280·1	483·5	799·4	1205·7	228·0	365·0
	65·1	66·1	62·5	66·2	76·6	83·9	89·0	85·1	80·6	99·5
1987	7·9	21·4	58·6	131·1	259·4	477·2	766·6	1193·6	218·4	355·1
	72·5	58·0	61·6	61·3	70·9	82·8	85·3	84·2	77·2	96·8
1988	8·0	19·6	50·0	125·8	240·6	434·8	751·6	1143·8	206·0	345·4
	73·4	53·1	52·6	58·8	65·8	75·4	83·6	80·7	72·8	94·1
1989	4·8	20·9	49·0	113·3	223·3	397·5	700·1	1094·7	190·4	335·8
	44·0	56·6	51·5	53·0	61·0	69·0	77·9	77·2	67·3	91·5

*WHO European standard population.

109

TABLE II—Mortality from coronary heart disease in England and Wales in women by age group and year. Mortality is expressed as rate per 100 000 and as percentages of rate in 1972

Year	Age group (years)									
	30-34	35-39	40-44	45-49	50-54	55-59	60-64	65-69	30-64*	Total
1972	2·1	5·5	14·6	33·3	66·6	135·8	272·2	515·7	65·9	254·8
1973	2·0	4·6	16·4	36·5	66·2	132·2	274·2	522·1	66·2	256·3
	95·2	83·6	112·3	109·6	99·4	97·4	100·1	101·2	100·5	100·6
1974	1·4	5·6	16·4	34·3	66·3	140·0	275·8	512·3	67·1	258·9
	66·7	101·8	112·3	103·0	99·6	103·1	101·3	99·3	101·8	101·6
1975	2·3	6·3	14·7	32·5	67·2	136·7	264·4	511·4	65·3	259·9
	109·5	114·6	100·7	97·6	100·9	100·7	97·1	99·2	99·1	102·0
1976	1·7	5·2	16·9	34·1	66·7	133·9	276·2	508·7	66·4	268·2
	80·9	94·6	115·8	102·4	100·2	98·6	101·5	98·6	100·8	105·3
1977	2·1	5·2	14·3	32·5	66·4	132·6	264·8	497·4	64·4	263·5
	100·0	94·6	98·0	97·6	99·7	97·6	97·3	96·5	97·8	103·4
1978	1·9	5·9	14·8	31·7	71·5	138·4	277·4	517·1	67·3	270·1
	90·5	107·3	101·4	95·2	107·4	101·9	101·9	100·3	102·2	106·0
1979	2·1	4·4	13·8	32·3	73·1	137·5	284·1	493·1	67·9	258·1
	100·0	80·0	94·5	97·0	109·8	101·3	104·4	95·6	103·1	101·3
1980	2·1	4·5	12·7	27·1	63·5	141·2	275·9	490·4	65·1	256·2
	100·0	81·8	87·0	81·4	95·4	104·0	101·4	95·1	98·9	100·6
1981	2·0	4·7	12·9	27·3	64·0	134·4	250·9	480·4	61·7	259·5
	95·2	85·5	88·4	82·0	96·1	99·0	92·2	93·2	93·7	101·8
1982	1·2	4·2	10·9	24·4	62·4	131·2	256·0	483·0	60·6	258·8
	57·1	76·4	74·7	73·3	93·7	96·6	94·1	93·7	92·0	101·6
1983	1·8	4·4	10·2	25·8	62·2	138·4	265·4	487·2	62·8	263·1
	85·7	80·0	69·9	77·5	93·4	101·9	97·5	94·5	95·3	103·3
1984	1·7	3·4	9·6	24·6	59·3	134·2	264·9	488·4	61·3	268·7
	85·7	61·8	65·8	73·9	89·0	98·8	97·3	94·7	93·1	105·5
1985	1·5	3·6	9·2	23·6	58·5	129·2	269·1	479·0	60·8	279·3
	71·4	65·5	63·0	70·9	87·8	95·1	98·9	92·9	92·3	109·6
1986	1·4	4·5	8·7	22·1	53·2	125·4	261·5	471·7	58·5	271·1
	66·7	81·8	59·6	66·4	79·9	92·3	96·1	91·5	88·8	106·4
1987	1·8	3·9	8·2	21·6	50·6	122·0	261·6	470·5	57·5	265·1
	85·7	70·9	56·2	64·9	76·0	89·8	96·1	91·2	87·3	104·0
1988	1·1	3·6	8·3	19·0	46·6	109·6	249·4	452·7	53·4	264·2
	52·4	65·5	56·9	57·1	70·0	80·7	91·6	87·8	81·1	103·7
1989	1·2	3·3	7·4	17·1	43·4	107·1	234·5	442·1	50·5	262·4
	57·1	60·0	50·7	51·4	65·2	78·9	86·2	85·7	76·7	103·0

*WHO European standard population.

the population in older age groups). For each year the mortality per 100 000 is followed by that rate as a percentage of the mortality in 1972. Table III shows the average annual decline in mortality over the 17 years since 1972 and for lesser intervals down to one year.

What this mass of figures reveals on close inspection is that the

TABLE III—Average annual percentage decline in mortality from coronary heart disease in men and women over different time intervals up to 1989

Period (years)	Age group (years)									
	30-34	35-39	40-44	45-49	50-54	55-59	60-64	65-69	30-64*	Total
Men										
17	3·3	2·6	2·9	2·8	2·3	1·8	1·3	1·3	1·9	0·5
12	4·0	2·8	3·7	3·3	3·1	2·5	1·7	1·7	2·5	0·8
10	5·2	3·1	3·9	4·0	3·8	3·2	2·4	1·8	3·2	1·1
5	7·8	1·1	4·3	5·0	4·4	4·8	3·1	2·9	4·1	1·7
3	10·8	4·8	5·8	6·7	6·8	5·9	4·1	3·1	5·5	6·6
2	19·6	1·2	8·2	6·8	7·0	8·4	4·3	4·1	6·4	2·7
1	40·0	+6·6	2·0	9·9	7·2	8·6	6·9	4·3	7·6	2·8
Women										
17	2·5	2·4	2·9	2·9	2·0	1·2	0·8	0·8	1·4	+0·2
12	3·6	3·0	4·0	3·9	2·9	1·6	1·0	0·9	1·8	0·0
10	4·3	2·5	4·6	4·7	4·1	2·2	1·7	1·0	2·6	+0·2
5	5·9	0·6	4·6	6·1	5·4	4·0	2·3	1·9	3·5	0·5
3	4·8	8·9	5·0	7·5	6·1	4·9	3·4	2·1	4·6	1·1
2	16·7	7·7	4·9	10·4	7·1	6·1	5·2	3·0	6·1	0·5
1	+9·1	8·3	10·8	10·0	6·9	2·3	6·0	2·3	5·4	0·7

*Who European standard population.

coronary mortality in England and Wales is well past its peak and that the climax was reached in different years in different age and sex groups. The decline apparently began earlier and has been greater in the younger age groups than the older ones, and in men rather than women. Rates in the youngest age groups are unstable from year to year because of the small numbers of deaths, and until mortality began to fall in those aged 55-64 the age standardised rate was almost unaffected. Within the past few years, however, the rate of decline has been substantial. In men the age standardised rate in each year has been lower than the previous one since 1978, and in women since 1983. In both sexes rates might now be said to be in free fall. Rates for men under 50 in 1989 are nearly half of those in 1972 while the age standardised rate for the age group 30-64 is down by a third.

Possible target

- 30% Reduction between 1988 and the year 2000 in the number of deaths from coronary heart disease in people under 65

The government's proposed target is for a 30% reduction in mortality over the 12 years from 1988 to the year 2000.[1] This means an annual average fall (neglecting compound interest) of 2·5%. An average annual decline of 2·5% certainly seems to be optimistic compared with the average change over 17 years. It equals the rate of change in men over the past 12 years and exceeds that in women. The rate of decline, however, has been accelerating, and compared with the rate of decline over the past 10 years, five years, three years, or two years a decline of 2·5% seems unduly conservative.

One sympathises with the secretary of state's advisers in suggesting a target that seems both credible and feasible, but 2·5% a year seems somewhat pessimistic. The same WHO statistical tables show that countries which began their decline earlier, such as the United States and Australia, have sustained rates of decline near to the 6% achieved in England and Wales in the past few years. Halving of the mortality from premature coronary heart disease not only would be a more striking target than 30%, but also seems reasonable and achievable if the current rate of improvement can be maintained. The 30% should be made 50%.

A mortality target does have the advantage of being based on routinely available death certificates, but it considers only the first of the three criteria for a disease problem. Death certificates are not necessarily subject to verification, and it leaves morbidity and economic cost aside. Though it would be attractive to target reduction in non-fatal myocardial infarction in parallel with mortality, there are probably two reasons why this was not done. Firstly, reports from countries in the vanguard of declining mortality are by no means unanimous in suggesting that non-fatal infarction follows the same trend as mortality. Secondly, special monitoring would be needed, something that needs to be set up and funded long term. Although the protocol for WHO's MONICA project (monitoring cardiovascular disease) was largely written in London[5] and the quality control centre for event registration is in Britain, the Department of Health in London decided in the early 1980s not to fund any participating centres in England and Wales, leaving Scotland and Northern Ireland to contribute data for the United Kingdom. Coronary event registration has been carried out according to different criteria for some years in Nottingham, but a morbidity target for coronary disease should ideally entail monitoring more than one English population and preferably would use an internationally standardised protocol. Monitoring of myocardial infarction poses one set of problems.

Monitoring angina pectoris (not included in the MONICA project), would pose another. Given the cost of angina pectoris to the NHS and its importance these problems ought to be looked at seriously.

What should the strategy for reaching the targets be?

The consultative document lists smoking, diet (including blood cholesterol concentration), physical fitness, and blood pressure as relevant risk factors that can be influenced. Each is considered as a separate key area and will be discussed as such by other commentators in this series of articles, so my comments will be brief and selective.

How much the decline in mortality from coronary heart disease is related to changes in the major known risk factors in England and elsewhere, and how much to factors unknown, remains controversial (and was the dilemma in the US that led to WHO's MONICA initiative in 1979.[5]). In general, however, declining mortality has been associated with improving risk factor levels. Hastening these improvements should benefit both individual people and populations.

Cigarette smoking is an avoidable factor. It is an addictive drug that kills, accounting for a large proportion of premature deaths from coronary disease. It should be recognised and treated as such. British ambivalence and mixed messages should end. Every encouragement should be given to smokers to stop while limiting their opportunities to smoke anywhere except as consenting adults in private. We should aim to raise a smoke free generation of teenagers (both in the active and passive sense) for the next century. It is inconceivable that tobacco advertising will be legal in Britain for much longer, though whether it is this government or a subsequent one that makes the inevitable decision remains to be seen. In Europe we seem to be dragging our feet.

The consultative document's comments on diet came out just before a report by the Committee on Medical Aspects of Food Policy.[6] Dietary trends in the middle class seem to be generally favourable, although dietary fat composition seems to be changing more than total consumption. This is probably contributed to by the poor average standard of nutrition labelling in Britain coupled with the tendency of the food industry to remove fat from foods where it is noticed and put it back into foods where it isn't. However, there are concerns about the nutrition of young people, a disproportionate percentage of whom are raised in low income households. Many home providers have no knowledge or training in cooking or nutrition, which does not figure in the core school curriculum, and there are no national nutritional standards for school meals. The educational gap is filled by commercial promotion of products with the greatest added value rather than those with greatest nutritional value.

British blood cholesterol concentrations are high by international standards,[7] and to set a target to lower them to current American values by the end of the century is reasonable. This could be achieved by a national nutrition policy rather than by mass cholesterol testing and drugs.[8] (Paradoxically, in view of the decline in mortality, what poor British data there are suggest that cholesterol concentrations have not changed in the past decade,[8-10] so they are not the engine of that decline, although other dietary changes may be.) Although diet is an immensely complex subject, what is encouraging is the large degree of congruence between the dietary recommendations for minimising the risk of several different disease problems.[11]

In exercise the problem is to change physical exertion from a competitive activity predicated on success in teenagers and young adults to a social activity for all mature adults, designed into the urban environment.

In the monitoring of coronary risk factors England has again suffered in comparison with Scotland and Northern Ireland by not participating in WHO's MONICA project.[57] This is generating international comparative and longitudinal data on risk factors and trends in defined communities, the first large scale results coming from the early to mid-1980s. This deficiency will now be remedied, albeit on small national population samples.

What are the problems in achieving the targets?

England has been late in attempting to set up a health strategy, having failed to respond to the WHO initiative[12] or to the American example,[13] for several years. The consultative document shows a significant change of attitude at the highest level in the Department of Health, whose attitude to such WHO initiatives in the past, and to British researchers involved in them, has not always been encouraging. However, these welcome strategy initiatives have to outlast the present secretary of state and the present government. They need to be endorsed and supported not only by professional groups, voluntary bodies, and public opinion but also by all the relevant government departments within Whitehall, some of which can make major decisions helping or harming the public health without it being in their remit to take it into account. Such decisions need to be coordinated at Cabinet level, as has been done in other countries and as was recommended first in the Canterbury report,[14] and subsequently by the National Forum for Coronary Heart Disease Prevention on several occasions.[15]

Other problems with the strategy relate to the different components of the United Kingdom and the degree to which decision making is delegated downwards to health regions and districts and upwards to the European Community. A health strategy and targets for England alone are complicated by the historical amalgamation of health statistics with Wales. Wales, Scotland, and Northern Ireland have a degree of autonomy in their health strategies. Because England is central and makes up the bulk of the United Kingdom it is difficult for the other three territories to operate entirely independently. Perhaps the recent appointment of the Scottish chief medical officer to the English post will help coordination

By the year 2000 the health strategies for different European states will need to be better coordinated and they will need consistently high standards of health monitoring to assess the impact of their single market policies on diverse populations. In the 1970s the European Commission seemed to be ignoring health and subsidising not only tobacco but almost all the agricultural products containing saturated fat. In the past few years some health initiatives from Brussels (which continues to subsidise tobacco production) have produced ambivalent or negative reactions from London, sometimes for doctrinaire reasons concerned with who decides. It is to be hoped that health promotion initiatives in England in the future will not be delayed just because other Europeans are enthusiastic.

Conclusion

Coronary heart disease is a major health problem that demands a powerful response. The target for reducing mortality from premature coronary heart disease by the year 2000 should be 50% and not 30%. Monitoring of morbidity should be instituted and appropriate targets developed. Monitoring of risk factors in England has been inadequate and was rightly criticised by the public accounts committee.[16 17] Current proposals for monitoring in England are welcome but inadequate to report what is happening to regional and social subgroups in an increasingly heterogeneous population. The establishment of strong national smoking and nutrition policies should be an urgent priority.

Tabulations of mortality for different countries from the 1950s were provided by WHO Geneva. The views expressed here are those of the author and not those of any funding body.

1 Secretary of State for Health. *The health of the nation*. London: HMSO, 1991. (Cm 1523.)
2 Health Education Authority. *Health update 1: coronary heart disease*. London: HEA, 1990.
3 World Health Organisation European Collaborative Group. Multifactorial trial in the prevention of coronary heart disease. 3. Incidence and mortality results. *Eur Heart J* 1983;4:141-7.
4 World Health Organisation. *World health statistics annual 1990*. Geneva: WHO, 1990.
5 WHO MONICA Project Principal Investigators (prepared by Tunstall-Pedoe H). The World Health Organisation MONICA project (monitoring trends and determinants in cardiovascular disease): a major international collaboration. *J Clin Epidemiol* 1988;41:105-14.
6 Panel on Dietary Reference Values of the Committee on Medical Aspects of Food Policy. *Report. Dietary reference values for food energy and nutrients for the United Kingdom*. London: HMSO, 1991. (Department of Health report on health and social subjects 41.)
7 WHO MONICA Project. *A worldwide monitoring system for cardiovascular diseases. World Health Statistics Annual 1989*. Geneva: WHO, 1989.
8 Tunstall-Pedoe H, Smith WCS, Tavendale R. Howoften-that-high graphs of serum cholesterol. Findings from the Scottish Heart Health and Scottish MONICA studies. *Lancet* 1989;i:540-2.
9 Thelle DS, Shaper AG, Whitehead TP, Bullock DG, Ashby D. Blood lipids in middle-aged British men. *Br Heart J* 1983;49:205-13.
10 Gregory J, Foster K, Tyler H, Wiseman M. The dietary and nutritional survey of adults. London: Office of Population Censuses and Surveys, 1990.
11 WHO Study Group. Diet, nutrition, and the prevention of chronic diseases. *WHO Tech Rep Ser* 1990;797.
12 World Health Organisation Regional Office for Europe. *Targets for health for all*. Copenhagen: WHO, 1985.
13 United States Department of Health and Human Services. *Promoting health/preventing disease: objectives for the nation*. Washington, DC: United States Government Printing Office, 1980.
14 Steering Committee (chairman Rose G.) *Coronary heart disease: plans for action. A report based on an interdisciplinary workshop conference held at Canterbury, 28-30 September 1983*. London: Pitman, 1984.
15 National Forum for Coronary Heart Disease Prevention. *Action in the UK 1984-1987*. London: Health Education Authority, 1988.
16 National Audit Office. *Report by the Comptroller and Auditor General. National Health Service: coronary heart disease*. London: HMSO, 1989. (House of Commons Paper 208.)
17 House of Commons Committee on Public Accounts. *Coronary heart disease. 26th Report, session 1988-89*. London: HMSO, 1989.

Importance of obesity

JOHN GARROW

Circulatory disease, cancers, and respiratory disease account for 21%, 26% and 5% respectively of years of life lost up to the age of 65 and 13%, 7%, and 6% respectively of NHS expenditure.[1] These are the three biggest causes of mortality and morbidity. Obesity contributes to deaths from all three of these causes and is also associated with other diseases (figure), which makes it a prime candidate for being recognised as a key area.

For two decades it has been the received wisdom among epidemiologists that obesity is not an independent risk factor for cardiovascular disease. The seven nations study showed that if you know the age, blood pressure, smoking habits, and serum cholesterol concentration of men aged 40-60 then knowing their adiposity does not help to make any better prediction about which men will have a heart attack in the next five years.[2] Even if this premise is correct (and other investigators have reached different conclusions from analysis of the same data[3]) it does not follow that obesity is benign—it has been called the most readily identifiable of all risk factors.[4]

How obesity causes disease

Recent work on obesity in animal models has shown that the primary metabolic defect is a reduced sensitivity to insulin, from which all the other metabolic characteristics associated with obesity follow.[5] The classic study by Sims et al showed that if experimental obesity is produced by prolonged overfeeding of normal men with no family history of diabetes a similar syndrome of insulin insensitivity is produced, which reverts to normal with weight loss.[6] Susceptibility to arterial disease increases in parallel with increasing glucose intoler-

117

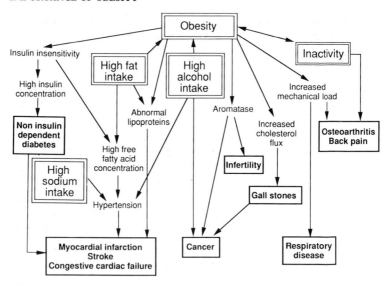

Effect of obesity and activities leading to obesity on important causes of death and illness

ance,[4] so this is one route by which obesity predisposes to cardio-vascular disease. Glucose intolerance, or serum insulin concentration, is also highly correlated with hypertension.[7] In addition, regardless of insulin insensitivity, obesity is associated with an unfavourable plasma lipoprotein pattern, with high low density lipoprotein cholesterol and triglyceride concentrations and low high density lipoprotein cholesterol concentration,[4 8] which is also linked with cardiovascular disease.

Another route by which obesity causes disease arises because adipose tissue contains the enzyme system aromatase, which converts androgens to oestrogens.[9] The resulting hormonal imbalance contributes to infertility and the polycystic ovary syndrome, which are common complications of obesity. The imbalance also probably explains the increased prevalence of sex hormone sensitive cancers in obese people.[10] Adipose tissue is also an important reservoir of cholesterol, so obese people have a greatly increased cholesterol flux and supersaturated bile,[11] which makes them prone to gall stones, abnormal liver function,[12] and gall bladder cancer.[10]

Finally, the increased mechanical load associated with obesity contributes to the reduced exercise tolerance and respiratory problems of obese people and the increased risk of musculoskeletal diseases and osteoarthritis in weight bearing joints.[9][13]

Does weight loss reverse the health risk of obesity?

Indirect evidence strongly suggests that weight loss does reverse almost all the health hazards of obesity. Life insurance data show that people who were impaired solely on account of obesity have normal insurance risks after losing weight.[14] The reversibility of insulin insensitivity has already been mentioned,[6] and all the risk factors for coronary heart disease—blood pressure; cholesterol, triglyceride, uric acid, and fasting glucose concentrations; forced vital capacity—also improve with weight loss.[15][16] The obese patient who loses weight is likely to improve greatly with respect to infertility[17] and osteoarthritis of the knees.[18] There is no information about the effect of weight loss on the risk of sex hormone sensitive cancers or on the social discrimination that obese people often suffer,[19] but from our knowledge of the aetiology it is reasonable to expect that these would also improve.

The only disadvantage of losing weight seems to be that while it is being lost the mobilisation of cholesterol in adipose tissue makes the bile even more saturated.

Case against obesity as key area

I have already considered and dismissed the fallacious argument that obesity by itself is not a risk factor. More serious objections are

---

Government's view on obesity

Obesity is increasing in both men and women. In 1986-7, 12% of women and 8% of men were obese compared with 8% and 6% respectively in 1980. In addition, 37% of men and 24% of women were overweight in 1986-7.

High blood cholesterol concentrations and raised blood pressure are linked with obesity. Both these conditions could be addressed by a reduction in obesity.

Target: By the year 2000 the proportion of obese adults should be 7% or less.

---

that obesity cannot be effectively treated, that campaigns against obesity will increase the prevalence of anorexia nervosa, and that obesity confers some protection against hip fracture in old people.

The effective treatment of obesity requires patience and an understanding of the principles of energy balance,[20] qualities which some doctors are unable or unwilling to deploy, so they declare obesity to be untreatable.[21] However, there is no metabolic barrier to achieving any desired weight loss with a conventional energy reducing diet[9 22]; the effectiveness of treatment depends mainly on the conviction of patient and therapist that weight loss is possible and worth the effort.

People who campaign against obesity need to be aware that any advice about how to lose weight will be avidly taken up by young women of normal weight who want to be unphysiologically thin. It is therefore necessary to specify clearly the range of weight for height for which the advice is given and to avoid concepts such as "an ideal weight"; instead, a range of desirable weights should be specified. There is no evidence that propaganda against obesity thus worded increases the prevalence of anorexia nervosa. Also such advice should be aimed chiefly at overweight young people (see below); old people benefit less and are disadvantaged more by weight loss.

Targets for preventing obesity

The target proposed by the Department of Health for obesity contains one prevalence for adults of all ages (box). The excess mortality associated with obesity is highest among people under 50 years old; those who will be 50 in 2005 are 36 years old now. I propose that the targets should be different for different age groups. The table shows the prevalence of obesity in the United Kingdom in 1980 and 1987 and my suggested targets for the year 2005.

Strategy to achieve targets

I believe that three components are needed for effective prevention of obesity in Britain. Firstly, the public must be informed about the range of weight for height that is associated with appreciable health risks in order to warn those who should be taking some action and to reassure those who should not. This is already being undertaken by the Health Education Authority,[24] but it is a task in which all health carers should share.

120

Prevalence (%) of obesity (Quetelet's index $>30\,kg/m^2$) in a representative sample of men and women aged 16-64 in the United Kingdom in 1980 and 1987[23] and target prevalences for the year 2005

Age (years)	Men			Women		
	1980	1987	2005	1980	1987	2005
16-24	2·5	3·0	2·0	3·5	6·0	2·0
25-34	4·5	6·0	4·0	4·5	11·0	4·0
35-49	8·0	11·0	6·0	9·9	10·0	6·0
50-64	7·7	9·0		14·3	18·0	

Secondly, there must be affordable slimming groups open to members of the public who want sound advice about dieting The information should go beyond the narrow objective of weight loss and should incorporate advice on intake of fats, alcohol, salt, and fibre[25] and on exercise.[26] Such a scheme has been running in the Harrow Health District for 14 years.[27] The members are mainly married women, who are well placed to pass on this information to their families. It greatly strengthens the authority of leaders of such groups if a specialist hospital clinic provides back up to cope with members who are "difficult" to help for metabolic or personality reasons.

Thirdly, there should be a policy in primary schools to identify children starting school who are above the 90th centile of weight for height and to provide facilities so these children increase normally in height between the ages of 7 and 12 years but slightly less than normally in weight. An average child gains about 22 kg over these five years, and a 7 year old who is 4 kg overweight for height is appreciably overweight. If that child gains 18 kg by the age of 12, he or she should then be normal weight for height.

Problems of implementing this strategy

There should be no great difficulty about implementing the first two components of the strategy; pilot schemes have been running well. But there has never been an organised attempt to prevent obesity in our schools, and this requires the intelligent cooperation of parents, school teachers, community dietitians, school nurses, and caterers. Unfortunately, giving overweight children fruit instead of sweets and low energy drinks instead of sugary colas may be seen as a punishment instead of an advantage. As always, education is the key, and rapid results are not to be expected.

This strategy also needs the backing of those in primary health care, who could easily sabotage the scheme by hostility or even indifference. We lack any systematic information about what general practitioners do for their obese patients and with what effect, and we do not know what proportion of practices regard obesity as a cosmetic problem for which the remedies are available from commercial slimming clinics. Research into this is urgently needed.

1 Secretary of State for Health. *The health of the nation*. London, HMSO, 1991. (Cm 1523.)
2 Keys A, Aravanis C, Blackburn H, van Buchem FSP, Buzina R, Djordjeuik BS, *et al*. Coronary heart disease: overweight and obesity as risk factors. *Ann Intern Med* 1972;**117**:15-27.
3 Hubert H. The importance of obesity in the development of coronary risk factors and disease: the epidemiological evidence. *Annu Rev Public Health* 1986;**7**:493-502.
4 Shaper AG. *Coronary heart disease, risks and reasons*. London: Current Medical Literature, 1988.
5 Jeanrenaud B. Neuroendocrinology and evolutionary aspects of experimental obesity. In: Oomura Y, Tarui S, Inoue S, Shimazu T, eds. *Progress in obesity research 1990*. London: John Libbey, 1991:409-21.
6 Sims EAH, Danforth EJr, Horton ES, Bray GA, Glennon JA, Salans LB. Endocrine and metabolic effects of experimental obesity in man. *Recent Prog Horm Res* 1973;**29**:457-96.
7 Modan M, Halkin H, Almog S, Lusky A, Eshkol A, Shefi M, *et al*. Hyperinsulinaemia: a link between hypertension obesity and glucose intolerance. *J Clin Invest* 1985;**75**:809-17.
8 Forde OH, Thelle DS, Arnesen E, Mjos OD. Distribution of high density lipoprotein cholesterol according to relative body weight, cigarette smoking and leisure time physical activity. *Acta Med Scand* 1986;**219**:167-71.
9 Garrow JS. *Obesity and related diseases*. London: Churchill Livingstone, 1988.
10 Garfinkel L. Overweight and cancer. *Ann Intern Med* 1985;**103**:1034-6.
11 Reuben A, Maton PN, Murphy GM, Dowling RH. Bile lipid secretion in obese and non-obese individuals with and without gall stones. *Clin Sci* 1985;**69**: 71-9.
12 Nomura F, Ohnishi K, Satomura Y, Ohtsuki T, Fukungaga K, Honda M, *et al*. Liver function in moderate obesity—study in 534 moderately obese subjects among 4613 male company employees. *Int J Obes* 1986;**10**:349-54.
13 Rissanen A, Heliovaara M, Knekt P, Reunanen A, Aromaa A, Maatela J. Risk of disability and mortality due to overweight in a Finnish population. *BMJ* 1990;**301**:835-6.
14 Dublin LI. Relation of obesity to longevity. *N Engl J Med* 1853;**248**:971-4.
15 Borkan GA, Sparrow D, Wisniewski C, Vokonas PS. Body weight and coronary heart disease risk: patterns of risk factor change associated with long-term weight change. *Am J Epidemiol* 1986;**124**:410-9.
16 Hubert HB, Feinleib M, McNamara PM, Castelli WP. Obesity as an independent risk factor for cardiovascular disease: a 26-year follow-up of participants in the Framingham heart study. *Circulation* 1983;**67**:968-77.
17 Friedman CI, Kim MH. Obesity and its effect on reproductive function. *Clin Obstet Gynecol* 1985;**28**:645-63.
18 Dixon AS, Henderson D. Prescribing for osteoarthritis. *Prescribers' Journal* 1973;**13**:41-9.
19 Sonne-Holm S, Sorensen TI. Prospective study of attainment of social class of severely obese subjects in relation to parents' social class, intelligence and education. *BMJ* 1986;**292**:586-9.
20 Garrow JS. Treating obesity. *BMJ* 1991;**302**:803-4.
21 Hall A, Stewart D. Obesity: time for sanity and humanity. *N Z Med J* 1989;**102**:134-6.
22 Bortz WM. A 500 pound weight loss. *Am J Med* 1969;**47**:325-31.
23 Gregory J, Foster K, Tyler H, Wiseman M. *The dietary and nutritional survey of adults*. London, HMSO, 1990.
24 Garrow JS. *Overweight and obesity: a briefing paper*. London: Health Education Authority (in press).
25 Bingham S. Dietary aspects of a health strategy for England. *BMJ* 1991;**303**: 353-5.
26 Pentecost BL. *Medical aspects of exercise*. London, Royal College of Physicians of London, 1991.
27 Bush A, Webster J, Chalmers G, Pearson M, Penfold P, Brereton P, *et al*. The Harrow Slimming Club: report on 1090 enrolments in 50 courses, 1977-1986. *Journal of Human Nutrition and Dietetics* 1988;**1**:429-36.

Alcohol as a key area

PETER ANDERSON

Alcohol satisfies the government's criteria for inclusion as a key area and should form part of a health strategy for England.[1] Alcohol consumption is a major cause of premature death and avoidable ill health in the whole population; effective interventions are possible for reducing alcohol consumption which offer significant scope for improvement in health. Objectives and targets related to alcohol consumption can be set, and progress towards them can be monitored.

Burden of ill health

The harms related to alcohol consumption are many and act at both population and individual levels.[2-5] They include physical ill health; psychological ill health; public disorder, violence, and crime; family disputes; child neglect and abuse; road traffic accidents; accidents at work and in the home; fire; drowning; and employment problems. The total costs of harm to society are difficult to estimate. Economic costs for the United Kingdom related to alcohol consumption are more than £2 billion annually,[6] and estimates of the deaths attributable to alcohol consumption in England and Wales vary from 5000 to 40 000.[7]

At population and individual levels as alcohol consumption increases harm increases and as consumption decreases so does harm. This is illustrated by what happened in the United Kingdom in 1981-2, when consumption of alcohol fell from 10·4 litres of pure alcohol per adult to 9·2 litres. The fall was associated with an 11% reduction in convictions for drunkenness, an 8% fall in drinking and driving convictions, and a 4% fall in deaths from liver cirrhosis.[8]

Setting and monitoring targets

Many different types of targets can be set. One target should relate to alcohol consumption. Because of tax and excise, routine national data are available for trade and production of alcohol from which alcohol consumption per person can be calculated.[9] Regular national surveys of drinking habits are provided by the general household survey[10] and ad hoc but frequent inquiries of drinking are undertaken by the Social Survey Division of the Office of Population Censuses and Surveys.[11] Other targets should relate to reducing risk, state of health, and provision of services.

Risk reduction

Changes in consumption affect drinkers at all levels of consumption. The mean alcohol consumption of a community and the prevalence of heavy drinking are highly correlated ($r=0.97$), such that a mean reduction of alcohol consumption of 10% would correspond with a fall of about 10% in the numbers of heavy drinkers.[12] A Scottish study showed that after a substantial rise in the price of alcoholic beverages in the 1981 budget heavy and problem drinkers reduced their consumption in parallel with more modest consumers.[13]

Although heavy drinkers have a higher proportion of problems than other drinkers the contribution of heavy drinkers to the total number of alcohol related problems in the country is small. Most alcohol related problems occur in large numbers of light and moderate drinkers, although only a small proportion of such drinkers have alcohol related problems.[14] Thus two possible strategies exist to reduce risk: to target preventive activity at those identified as being heavy drinkers (the high risk approach) or to attempt to reduce consumption across the whole population.

The high risk approach is concerned with identifying and helping minorities with special problems by treating their risk factors or seeking changes in their behaviour. The aim is to truncate the risk distribution related to alcohol consumption, eliminating the high tail but not interfering with the rest of the population.[15] In practice, however, such truncation proves hard or impossible to achieve.

A population strategy has considerable advantages over the high risk approach. Firstly, the potential for reducing harm is greater.[14] Secondly, a population approach would aim at changing the perception of what are normal drinking levels and such a change would have

124

important consequences. An environment in which light drinking is the norm would exert a powerful pressure on people who drink heavily to reduce their consumption and so potentiate the high risk strategy.

Nevertheless, prevention measures that bring much benefit to the population in aggregate offer little to each participating individual and may result in poor motivation to reduce drinking on health grounds. A high risk approach may be needed to complement the population strategy, although by itself it is not sufficient.

Targets for alcohol consumption

The steady rise in alcohol consumption seen in this country since the 1950s seems to have been tailing off in the 1980s with a consumption per person of 9·6-9·8 litres a year (figure). An appropriate target might be that for people aged over 15 years consumption of pure alcohol per person should fall to 7·0 litres a year by the year 2000. In 1987 the level was 9·8 litres a year.[16] The target requires a fall in consumption of 28·6% and would bring alcohol consumption down to the level in the late 1960s.

One in four men and one in 12 women consume more than 21 and 14 standard units of alcohol a week respectively. A fall in overall consumption of 28% would automatically lead to a fall in the proportion of heavy drinkers of 28%.[12] Because service provision and education campaigns are targeted at reducing alcohol consumption among high risk drinkers higher targets for the fall in the proportions of men and women consuming more than currently recommended sensible levels could be achieved. Thus the government's target that by the year 2005 the number of men drinking more than 21 units a week should be no more than one in six and the number of women drinking more than 14 units a week no more than one in 18 could be achieved by the year 2000.

Improved health

Liver cirrhosis—The most important indicator of health for alcohol consumption is liver cirrhosis. Correlations between alcohol consumption and liver cirrhosis lie between 0·8 and 0·9. A fall in alcohol consumption of 28% would lead almost immediately to a fall in the death rate from cirrhosis and other chronic liver disease combined. Though there would be some latency in death rates from cirrhosis and a proportion of deaths are not caused by alcohol, improved treatment could decrease the death rates.[17] Thus a target to reduce the death rate

125

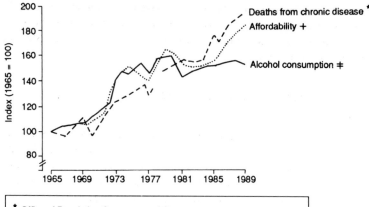

Alcohol consumption, affordability (personal disposable income/price of alcohol), and deaths from chronic liver disease. United Kingdom, 1965-89[1]

from cirrhosis by 28%, the same as alcohol consumption, would be feasible. In 1988 mortality from cirrhosis and other chronic liver disease combined was 55 per million population. This should be reduced to 40 per million population by the year 2000.

Road traffic accidents—Deaths from road traffic accidents and the number of such deaths related to alcohol are falling. In 1988 the figure was estimated to be 840. Assuming that the existing trend will continue, the target could be that by the year 2000 the number of deaths from road traffic accidents related to alcohol should be below 500.

Improved services and protection

Services should be based on primary health care with a partnership with specialist services.[18] Advice on screening, risk assessment, and intervention at a primary health care level is available. Interventions at a general practice level reduce alcohol consumption and are as effective as and cheaper than specialist treatment.[19 20] The first stage is for general practitioners to record alcohol consumption, and the target for the year 2000 should be that 95% of people aged over 18 years should have a general practitioner health record which includes alcohol consumption. I surveyed 20 000 medical records among 20 general practices within the Oxford region in 1989 and found that only 7% of notes contained a dated record of a quantitative measure of alcohol consumption.

Strategies for achieving the targets

National action

The most important determinant of alcohol consumption is affordability, as measured by personal disposable income divided by the price of alcohol (figure). As affordability increases so does consumption and vice versa. The price of alcohol can be manipulated by tax. Differential changes in tax for different alcoholic beverages in Britain have provided clear evidence of the importance of tax in determining alcohol consumption. Over the past 20 years the prices for spirits and wines have dropped more than 50% relative to income whereas prices of beers have dropped by only 16%. Over this period the proportion of total alcohol consumed as beer has fallen from 74% to 55% and the proportion of alcohol consumed as wines and spirits increased from 24% to 40%. Alcohol consumption could be reduced by manipulating the price of alcohol in relation to personal disposable income through taxation policy.[21]

Licensing laws are a second strategy by which alcohol consumption can be influenced nationally. Licensing laws are designed to limit or control the availability of alcohol. But changing the number of retail outlets for alcohol may affect consumption only in communities with few such outlets relative to the population. Consumption of alcohol rose by almost 50% in Finland in 1969 as a result of the 1968 Alcohol Act, which permitted the establishment of state alcohol shops and licensed restaurants in rural areas. In 1968 medium strength beer could be bought in 132 state alcohol shops and 911 restaurants, nearly all of which were in cities and towns. In 1969 there were 18 000 off premises outlets and 4000 on premises outlets for medium strength beer, nationwide.[22] The effect of restrictions in a country where alcohol retail outlets are already common has been calculated as a decrease of 2% in alcohol consumed for a 1% decrease in the number of licensed premises.[5]

Local action

National policy needs to be supported by local action. Indeed local action may help set the agenda for national policy. Broad based community multisectoral programmes are the key to achieving community wide changes in lifestyle and support for programmes managing the sale and use of alcohol.[23] That such programmes are successful is shown by the impact of a promotional campaign on the intention to comply with a policy to manage alcohol in the municipally owned recreation facilities in Thunder Bay, Ontario, Canada.[24] The policy, which was introduced in three stages from May 1980 to October 1982, recommended that alcohol be regulated so that alcohol consumption was not permitted in some recreational facilities, was limited to special occasions in other facilities, and to fully licensed use in still further facilities. A publicity campaign promoting the policy ran from May to July 1983. The impact of the policy on attitudes towards legal controls of alcohol was studied. The attitudes of the experimental group in Thunder Bay became less liberal while those of the control community did not change. This suggested that the promotional campaign had the effect of making people in Thunder Bay more receptive to the idea of managing the sale and use of alcohol.

Primary care services

Primary care is an important setting for identifying people at risk from heavy drinking and assisting them in reducing alcohol consumption. A high risk strategy based on primary health care can complement a national and local population based strategy. Primary health care has been shown to be effective and efficient. Intervention at the

---

Central policy review staff recommendations on alcohol

The government should announce a positive commitment to counter the rise in consumption of alcohol to reduce alcohol related disabilities.

The approach should be interpreted widely. It should influence alcohol policies in general and not only those concerned with the health consequences of misuse.

Trends towards making drink cheaper by not increasing revenue duties should be stopped. As a minimum duty should be kept in line with the retail price index

---

primary care level leads to reductions of alcohol consumption of around 15% and reductions in proportions of excessive drinkers of around 20% and cost one twentieth of the cost of specialist services.[25]

Problems in achieving targets

National level

Central government—The government needs to accept that it has a legitimate role in determining and implementing policy related to alcohol consumption. This was most clearly stated in the 1979 report by the central policy review staff, which was never published.[26] The first three items of a seven point programme outlined in the report's recommendations are given in the box.

The alcohol industry is large, well established, and powerful. In 1986-7, tax revenue from alcoholic drinks sales was £6447 million and in 1987 the industry provided jobs for over 1 million people.[21] The industry's structure is such that a few firms control most of the market—for example, 80% of the market share for beer is divided between just six companies. This allows the industry to take a consistent position and to lobby the government with considerable success. However, it should also allow negotiation of a common approach towards policies for the marketing and distribution of a product which causes society not only harm but also some benefit. National negotiation is complicated by the internationalisation of the industry. The advent of an open European market in 1992 will compound the difficulties of dealing with the industry nationally. Furthermore, the increasing corporatism of large industries with the industry having interdependent ties with other corporate interests results in an ownership structure of such complexity that it is difficult to identify a simple set of alcohol industry owners.

Public awareness needs to be increased, particularly the understanding of the need to change the population distribution of alcohol consumption rather than target high risk drinkers. Current education campaigns which focus on sensible levels of drinking may be counterproductive to this population based approach.

Local action

The main impediment to adoption and implementation of local alcohol policies and strategies is the will and the perception that something can be done. Every local community, however, has largely untapped preventive services which can be mobilised. Means of

129

achieving this include disseminating examples of good practice and providing resources to maintain programmes once adopted.

Action at the primary health care level and the introduction of the new general practitioner contract will support the implementation of a health strategy for England. The adoption of national targets for a health strategy will need to be complemented by the adoption of general practice based targets for activity and outcome.

Conclusion

Alcohol is an important cause of death and ill health in the United Kingdom. The risk associated with alcohol consumption can be reduced by adopting national and local population based policies that are supported by risk reduction initiatives based in primary health care. The adoption of targets can be monitored and if implemented a health strategy incorporating alcohol as a key area will go some way towards improving the health of the nation.

1 Secretary of State for Health. *Health of the nation*. London: HMSO, 1991. (Cm 1523.)
2 Royal College of General Practitioners. *Alcohol—a balanced view*. London: Royal College of General Practitioners, 1986. (Reports from General Practice 24.)
3 Royal College of Psychiatrists. *Alcohol—our favourite drug*. London: Tavistock, 1986.
4 Royal College of Physicians. *A great and growing evil. The medical consequences of alcohol abuse*. London: Tavistock, 1987.
5 Faculty of Public Health Medicine. *Alcohol and the public health*. Basingstoke: Macmillan, 1991.
6 Robinson D, Maynard A, Chester R. *Controlling legal addictions*. London: Macmillan, 1989.
7 Anderson P. *Excess mortality associated with alcohol consumption*. BMJ 1988;**297**:824-6.
8 Kendell RE. The beneficial consequences of the United Kingdom's declining per capita consumption of alcohol in 1979-82. *Alcohol Alcohol* 1984;**19**: 271-6.
9 Spring JA, Buss DH. Three centuries of alcohol in the British diet. *Nature* 1977;**270**:567–72.
10 Office of Population Censuses and Surveys. *General household surveys*. London: HMSO, 1975-90.
11 Goddard E. *Drinking in England and Wales in the late 1980's*. London: HMSO, 1991.
12 Rose G, Pay S. The population mean predicts the number of deviant individuals. *BMJ* 1990;**301**:1031-4.
13 Kendell RE, De Romanie M, Ritson B. Effect of economic changes on Scottish drinking habits, 1978-1982. *Br J Addict* 1983;**78**:365-79.
14 Kreitman N. Alcohol consumption and the preventive paradox. *Br J Addict* 1986;**81**:353-63.
15 Rose G. Sick individuals and sick populations. *Int J Epidemiol* 1985;**14**:32-8.
16 Central Statistical Office. *Social trends*. No 20. London: HMSO, 1990.
17 Mann RE, Smart RG, Rush BR. Are decreases in liver cirrhosis rates a result of increased treatment for alcoholism. *Br J Addict* 1988;**83**:683-8.
18 Anderson P. *Management of drinking problems*. Copenhagen: World Health Organisation Regional Office for Europe, 1991.
19 Drummond DC, Thorn B, Brown C, Edwards G, Mullan MJ. Specialist versus general practitioner treatment of problem drinkers. *Lancet* 1990;**336**:915-8.
20 Potamianes G, North WRC, Meade TW, Townsend J, Peters TJ. Randomised trial of community based centre versus conventional hospital management in treatment of alcoholism. *Lancet* 1986;ii:797-9.
21 Maynard A, Tether P, eds. *Preventing alcohol and tobacco problems*. Vol 1. Aldershot: Avebruy, 1990.

22 Osterberg E. *Alcohol policy measures and the consumption of alcoholic beverages in Finland, 1950-1975.* Helsinki: Finnish Foundations for Alcohol Studies, 1980.

23 Giesbrecht N, ed. *Research, action and the community: experiences in the prevention of alcohol and other drug problems.* Washington, DC: US Government Printing Office, 1989.

24 Gliksman L, Thomson M, Moffatt K, Douglas K, Smythe C, Caverson R. *The impact of a promotional campaign on a community's intention to comply with a policy to manage alcohol in its municipally owned recreational facilities.* Toronto: Addiction Research Foundation, 1987. (Internal document 82.)

25 Anderson P. Primary care physicians and alcohol. *J R Soc Med* (in press).

26 Central Policy Review Staff. *Alcohol policies, 1979.* Stockholm: Sociologiska Institution, 1982.

Role of diabetes

K G M M ALBERTI

The Health of the Nation[1] is ostensibly a consultative document, but in the past such documents have been taken on as established policy all too rapidly. The document is none the less to be welcomed as it shows, firstly, a welcome move from administrative and financial priorities to real health issues and, secondly, a clear indication that prevention is to be targeted rather than disease. Sixteen key areas of interest have been chosen. The sting in the tail, however, is that only a few of these will be targeted initially. The criteria for final selection are, sadly, likely to be largely financial as well as health oriented, and payment for any new ventures will inevitably be at the expense of other aspects of health care or come out of so called "cost improvements." Below I present the case for and against including diabetes in the final list and discuss suggested targets and the strategy needed to achieve those targets.

Should diabetes be included?

The main criteria for selecting key areas are that the area should be a major cause of avoidable ill health, that effective interventions should be possible, and that it should be possible to set objectives and targets and monitor progress. Diabetes meets all these criteria.

The known prevalence of diabetes is about 0·3% for insulin dependent diabetes and 0·7% for non-insulin dependent diabetes.[2] A known prevalence of about 1% does not at first seem important when compared with other targeted conditions such as ischaemic heart disease and cancer. But 1% is undoubtedly an underestimate. It has been estimated that for every known person with non-insulin dependent diabetes there is another undiagnosed. Hence the real figure is closer to 2%, or 1 million diabetic people in England and Wales. With the increase in screening programmes in primary health care more of these unknown cases will inevitably be picked up. The numbers magnify in certain high risk groups.[3] For example, the prevalence of non-insulin dependent diabetes increases with age: 5-10% of those over 70 years will have the disorder. With the increase in the proportion of elderly people in the population the total prevalence of diabetes will also increase. Similarly certain immigrant groups such as Afro-Caribbeans and Asian Indians have overall prevalences of 5-10%.[4] Those with hypertension, heart disease, dyslipidaemia, and obesity are also more likely to have diabetes.

Long term complications

The striking feature of diabetes is the risk of developing long term complications: nephropathy, retinopathy, and neuropathy together with macroangiopathy. Overt nephropathy develops 10 to 20 years after the onset of insulin dependent diabetes[5] and five to 15 years after the onset of non-insulin dependent diabetes, the shorter time in the second type probably reflecting the delay in diagnosing non-insulin dependent diabetes in many people. Clinical nephropathy develops in only about a fifth of those with insulin dependent diabetes and fewer of those with non-insulin dependent diabetes, although incipient nephropathy, reflected by microalbuminuria, is more common.[6 7] The importance of the nephropathy lies in the progress to end stage renal failure and the consequent need for continuous ambulatory peritoneal dialysis or renal transplantation, or both. Diabetes is now one of the major causes of renal failure, particularly in younger subjects.[8] This results in a large social, personal, and economic burden.

Retinopathy eventually develops in most patients with diabetes of both forms. In most patients, however, only background retinopathy develops, which generally does not impair vision. Proliferative retinopathy, particularly in insulin dependent diabetes can cause blindness, and it makes diabetes the commonest cause of blindness in people under the age of 60 in Britain.[9] Patients with non-insulin dependent diabetes are particularly prone to develop maculopathy, again with serious impact on vision. There is also an increased risk of cataract.

Neuropathy, both somatic and autonomic, also occurs in diabetic patients. This has particular effects on legs and feet. Sensation is diminished, and this can lead to ulceration and, generally in combination with peripheral vascular disease, gangrene and the need

133

for amputation. Finally, macrovascular disease in the form of ischaemic heart disease, stroke, and peripheral vascular disease is two to five times more common in diabetic patients than in the general population and, indeed, is the main cause of premature death in diabetes.[10]

Acute complications

Diabetic patients may also have acute complications. Diabetic ketoacidosis is an important cause of death in diabetic subjects aged under 50[11] and mortality rises sharply with age.[12] Hypoglycaemia is also common, particularly in insulin dependent diabetes. Mild hypoglycaemia occurs with monotonous regularity, on average one episode every two weeks, whereas episodes requiring admission to hospital occur at a rate of 0·1 admission per patient year.[13] Even mild chronic hypoglycaemia may cause subtle neurological damage. Recently there has been emphasis on young patients dying of nocturnal hypoglycaemia—the "dead in bed" syndrome—which is rare but important as it occurs in young people.[14] In addition, hypoglycaemia is almost certainly much commoner than previously thought in non-insulin dependent diabetic patients taking sulphonylureas and contributes to confusional states in elderly people. Poorly controlled diabetes also increases susceptibility to infection.

Diabetes of both types is thus an important cause of morbidity and death. The economic costs of diabetes are about 5% of total NHS expenditure.[1] This excludes the costs to families of helping look after their diabetic relatives and the costs to the country of lost productivity. The key question is therefore whether diabetes represents a major cause of avoidable ill health.

Possibilities for preventing diabetes

Can ill health from diabetes be prevented? This can be considered on three fronts: primary prevention (Can diabetes itself be prevented?); secondary prevention (Even if diabetes occurs can the consequences be prevented?); and tertiary prevention (When the complications occur can morbidity and death from these be avoided?).

The Health of the Nation is remarkably vague on these issues, and indeed gives little attention to primary prevention. Insulin dependent diabetes is predominantly an autoimmune disease, and current work suggests that remission can be induced in some patients with drugs such as cyclosporin if they are started within six weeks of clinical

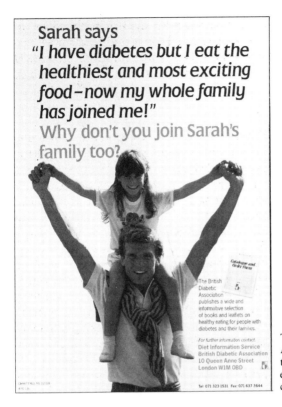

Sarah says "I have diabetes but I eat the healthiest and most exciting food – now my whole family has joined me!" Why don't you join Sarah's family too?

The British Diabetic Association publishes a wide and informative selection of books and leaflets on healthy eating for people with diabetes and their families.

For further information contact:
Diet Information Service
British Diabetic Association
10 Queen Anne Street
London W1M 0BD

Tel: 071 323 1531 Fax: 071 637 3644

The British Diabetic Association recognises the importance of education in preventing complications

presentation.[15] More specific drugs are needed, but when these are developed genuine preventive approaches can be tried by identifying patients during the long prodromal period of the disorder. Prevention of non-insulin dependent diabetes is probably more important in overall public health terms. As mentioned in the consultative document the condition is associated with obesity. Equally important is its strong association with physical inactivity.[16 17] Both of these are theoretically amenable to changes in lifestyle. In the long term more emphasis must be given to primary prevention as the only truly effective way to deal with the disorder.

Currently secondary prevention represents the main method of attack. Certainly the acute complications are avoidable, largely through education. Avoiding the long term complications is more difficult. The green paper baldly states that "blood glucose must be controlled and maintained within normal levels." This is over-simplistic. Although much indirect evidence supports the view that

135

such an approach will prevent the development of the specific complications, the results of two long term trials currently under way, the diabetes control and complications trial in insulin dependent diabetes[18] and the United Kingdom prospective diabetes study in non-insulin dependent diabetes,[19] are required to provide definitive proof. It is not known, for example, precisely what the threshold of blood glucose concentration is; normoglycaemia may not be necessary. It is also not known why some people never develop the complications despite poor glycaemic control. Moreover, there is no good evidence that glycaemic control is related to the main killer in diabetes, macrovascular disease. To prevent macrovascular disease efforts are needed to attack the known risk factors such as smoking, hypertension, dyslipidaemia, obesity, and physical inactivity that often accompany diabetes, particularly the non-insulin dependent form.[20]

Despite these caveats it should be emphasised that effective interventions are available. For non-insulin dependent diabetes diet forms the cornerstone of therapy, with a "healthy diet" aimed at maintaining a normal body mass index being the ideal. Exercise is also valuable when possible. Drugs such as sulphonylureas and metformin are also helpful when diet fails and insulin is of course also available. In insulin dependent diabetes insulin is indispensable. It is effective in that near normoglycaemia can be obtained, particularly with multiple daily injections, which have been eased by the availability of injection pens. None the less, absolute normalisation of metabolism is rarely achieved, partly because of the non-physiological injection route and partly because of the variability of absorption of insulin and imperfections of available insulins.[21] All these treatments are greatly aided by self monitoring of blood glucose concentration. In general, certainly by comparison with many other disorders, effective intervention is available for most patients, although further developments are needed.

Tertiary prevention is also relevant and possible. Sight threatening retinopathy can be treated effectively with laser therapy. The progress of nephropathy to end stage renal failure can be slowed by meticulous attention to control of blood pressure and a low protein diet. Neuropathy is more problematical, but it has been shown that amputation rates can be decreased considerably through good chiropody and education.[22] Less has been achieved for stroke and myocardial infarctions, although measures applicable to non-diabetic patients, such as stopping smoking and treatment of dyslipidaemia and hypertension, will be just as important if not more important in the diabetic person.

Overall the balance is undoubtedly in favour of diabetes being included as a key area. It is a clearly defined condition with serious long term sequelae which have a major impact on up to 1 million people and, inevitably, their friends and families as well as being a high cost to the NHS. In addition, by contrast with almost every other suggested key area care of diabetic patients is discrete, definable, and organised. There is an active patient organisation with more than 140 000 members (the British Diabetic Association). Every district has a diabetes service, and all but 17 have a specialist diabetologist. Diabetes liaison nurses are widespread and minimum requirements for care have been established.[23] Diabetes has been targeted by general practice as a major area of interest, and WHO Europe is leading a campaign to diminish the adverse health impact of diabetes. The Royal College of Physicians is coordinating the production of management protocols and, together with the diabetic association and the King's Fund, is examining audit and outcome measures. The Department of Health has already funded a study into the cost effectiveness of different methods of screening for retinopathy.[24] There is thus already considerable activity and a powerful infrastructure is in place; this should allow the easy transition of diabetes into a key area for action under the government's strategy.

Setting targets

Targets are obviously needed. One set was produced in 1989 at a meeting organised by WHO Europe and the European region of the International Diabetes Federation: the St Vincent Declaration.[25] Some of these are quoted in the consultative document (box). They suffer in part by being stated as proportional rather than absolute changes. None the less, these are reasonable aims. The consultative document, however, states that we do not have the baseline information, so that it is not possible to monitor the targets. This is a typical negative approach. It should be possible to establish rather quickly the numbers of diabetic patients going blind; requiring laser therapy; developing end stage renal failure; or having amputations, strokes, peripheral vascular disease, and heart attacks in targeted health regions if not in the whole country.

The government also suggests some proxy targets (box). The target relating to free eye tests for diabetic patients is a little odd as most diabetic clinics already screen for retinopathy with a camera or by direct funduscopy. These proxies are a little woolly in concept and are in danger of confusing process with outcome, although good practice in process is likely to aid outcome. There are other possible short term targets which should be included such as numbers of admissions to hospital for diabetes related causes; average glycaemic control; and proportion of patients reviewed in hospital or general practice a minimum number of times a year.

Overall it would seem wise to adopt the St Vincent Declaration, which includes many other suggestions relating to education and training, in the first place and to capitalise on the rapid progress being made by the St Vincent Declaration working group in the production of protocols, guidelines, and, in particular, standard computerised records. The criterion of setting challenging but achievable targets that can be monitored though appropriate indicators can certainly be met for diabetes, although further work in the short term will be needed.

Strategy for reaching the targets

The key to reaching the targets is improvement in the organisation of care. Much groundwork has already been done, and the minimum requirements for diabetes care in hospital based services have been published.[23]

Proposals for general practice based care are less clear, and there is a real danger that some patients will be kept in general practice and not receive optimal or even minimal care because of the new funding arrangements. Nevertheless, it should be possible for district diabetes committees, which already exist in many regions, to agree on establishing a district register, protocols, minimum standards, audit concepts, etc.

Barriers to achievement

The major problem is finance. If more diabetic patients are found and those currently receiving little or no care start to receive appropriate care the patient load will increase by 50% or more. More staff will be required, particularly diabetes nurse specialists and dietitians for education. We are also well short of the previously stated target of one diabetologist per 100 000 population.[23] We will also need more chiropodists, better eye screening facilities, and more capacity

Targets suggested by government for diabetes

The government would welcome views on the feasibility of adopting the targets agreed in the St Vincent Declaration:

- To reduce new blindness due to diabetes by one third or more
- To reduce by one half the rate of limb amputation for diabetic gangrene
- To achieve a pregnancy outcome in diabetic women similar to that of non-diabetic women
- To reduce the numbers of people entering end stage diabetic renal failure by at least one third
- To cut morbidity and mortality from coronary heart disease in people with diabetes by vigorous programmes of risk factor reduction.

Additionally, it is known that certain service activities are likely to produce good health outcomes. Until the information becomes available to use the outcome measures in the St Vincent Declaration service activities could be measured as a proxy for health outcomes.

Examples are:

- The proportion of general practices within a family health services authority area that follow protocols agreed locally between hospital clinicians and primary care staff for providing services to people with diabetes
- The proportion of people with diabetes screened, within a given period, for the long term complications of diabetes
- The proportion of people with diabetes who have received a free NHS eye test in the preceding year.

(This should eventually be superseded in time by a specific diabetic retinopathy screening programme for all those at high risk.)

to deal with renal failure and sight threatening retinopathy. Audit and measurement, recording, and assessment of outcomes will also consume resources. In the long term there will be savings, but with current methods of health service funding only short term expenditure is taken into account. A real increase in available funds will be needed; already staff cuts have been threatened in hospital based services for financial reasons and on the spurious grounds that diabetes is a primary health care disorder.

Other problems exist. Diabetes registers are needed throughout the country and will take time to establish. District policies need to be agreed and decisions made about which patients should be cared for in which setting. Monitoring of general practice and hospital services will be needed to ensure that minimum standards are being met. None of these problems are insurmountable provided that resources are available, and this must be the biggest question mark.

Conclusion

Diabetes is an excellent example of a chronic disorder for which preventive measures have an important role in long term outcome. It is an increasing problem, with at least 1 million people affected, and a major cause of blindness, renal failure, amputation, and premature cardiovascular disease. It fulfils all the criteria set down for inclusion as a key area. New resources will, however, be needed if the stated objectives are to be met.

1 Secretary of State for Health. *The health of the nation*. London: HMSO, 1991. (Cm 1523.)
2 Neil HAW, Gatling W, Mather HM, Thompson AV, Thorogood M, Fowler GH, *et al.* The Oxford community diabetes study: evidence for an increase in the prevalence of known diabetes in Great Britain. *Diabetic Med* 1987;4:539-43.
3 Williams DRR. Hospital admissions of diabetic patients: information from Hospital Activity Analysis. *Diabetic Med* 1985;2:27-32.
4 Mather HM, Keen H. The Southall diabetes survey: prevalence of known diabetes in Asians and Europeans. *BMJ* 1985;291:1081-4.
5 Andersen AR, Christiansen JS, Andersen JK, Kreiner S, Deckert T. Diabetic nephropathy in type 1 (insulin-dependent) diabetes: an epidemiological study. *Diabetologia* 1983;25:496-501.
6 Mogensen CE. Diabetic renal involvement and disease in patients with insulin-dependent diabetes. In: Alberti KGMM, Krall LP, eds. *Diabetes annual*. 4th ed. Amsterdam: Elsevier, 1988:411-48.
7 Marshall SM, Alberti KGMM. Comparison of the prevalence and associated features of abnormal albumin excretion in insulin-dependent and non-insulin-dependent diabetes. *Q J Med* 1989;261:61-71.
8 Working Party Report. Renal failure in the UK: deficient provision of care in 1985. *Diabetic Med* 1988;5:79-84.
9 Cullinan TR. Diabetic retinopathy and visual disability. *Diabetologia* 1982;23: 504-6.
10 Marks HH, Krall LP. Onset, course, prognosis and mortality in diabetes mellitus. In: Marbel A, White P, Bradley RF, Krall LP, eds. *Joslin's diabetes mellitus*. 11th ed. Philadelphia: Lea and Febiger, 1971:209-54.
11 Tunbridge WMG. Factors contributing to deaths of diabetics under fifty years of age. *Lancet* 1981;ii:569-72.
12 Gale EAM, Dornan TL, Tattersall RB. Severely uncontrolled diabetes in the over fifties. *Diabetologia* 1981;21:25-8.
13 Potter J, Clarke P, Gale EAM, Dave SH, Tattersall RB. Insulin-induced hypoglycaemia in an accident and emergency department: the tip of an iceberg. *BMJ* 1982;285:1180-2.

14 Campbell IW. Dead in bed syndrome: a new manifestation of nocturnal hypoglycaemia. *Diabetic Med* 1991;8:3-4.

15 Canadian-European Diabetes Study Group. Cyclosporin-induced remission of IDDM after early intervention: association of 1 year of cyclosporin treatment with enhanced insulin secretion. *Diabetes* 1988;37:1574-82.

16 Dowse GK, Zimmet PZ, Gareeboo H, Alberti KGMM, Tuomilehto J, Finch CF, *et al.* Abdominal obesity and physical inactivity are risk factors for both NIDDM and impaired glucose tolerance in Indian, Creole and Chinese Mauritians. *Diabetes Care* 1991;14:271-82.

17 Helmrich SP, Ragland DR, Leung RW, Paffenbarger RS. Physical activity and reduced occurrence of non-insulin-dependent diabetes mellitus. *N Engl J Med* 1991;325:147-52.

18 DCCT Research Group. Diabetes control and complications trial (DCCT): results of feasibility study. *Diabetes Care* 1987;10:1-19.

19 Multicentre Study Group. UK prospective study of therapies of maturity-onset diabetes. 1. Effect of diet, sulphonylurea, insulin or biguanide therapy on fasting plasma glucose and body weight over one year. *Diabetologia* 1983;24:404-11.

20 Reaven GM. Role of insulin resistance in human disease. *Diabetes* 1988;37: 1595-607.

21 Home PD, Thow JC. Insulin therapy. In: Alberti KGMM, Krall LP, eds. *Diabetes annual.* 6th ed. Amsterdam: Elsevier (in press).

22 Miller LV, Godstein J. More efficient care of diabetic patients in a county-hospital setting. *N Engl J Med* 1972;286:1388-91.

23 Royal College of Physicians and British Diabetic Association. *The provision of medical care for adult diabetic patients in the United Kingdom (1984).* London: Royal College of Physicians of London, 1985.

24 Sculpher MJ, Buxton MJ, Ferguson BA, Humphreys JE, Altman JFB, Spiegelhalter DJ, *et al.* A relative cost-effectiveness analysis of different methods of screening for diabetic retinopathy. *Diabetic Med* 1991;8:644-50.

25 World Health Organisation Europe and European Region of International Diabetes Federation. *The St Vincent Declaration.* Copenhagen: WHO Europe and the European Region of IDF, 1989.

HAROLD BRIDGES LIBRARY
S. MARTIN'S COLLEGE
LANCASTER

141

Strategy for a healthy environment

FIONA GODLEE

In *The Health of the Nation* diabetes and heart disease get six pages, prevention of accidents four, and the environment two.[1] This is not so bad. Other important health issues have, as this series has shown, been omitted from the document altogether. But the number of pages devoted to the environment, and its relegation to the back of the book, suggest either that the government does not perceive it to be a major influence on the nation's health or that it is not an area that lends itself to the setting of targets.

For some aspects of the environment these conclusions might be justified. It is, for example, difficult to establish that the failure of our drinking water to conform to European Community standards constitutes a real threat to health.[2] There are, however, other aspects of the environment—urban air pollution is one—where evidence of real harm does exist,[3] where large numbers of people are affected, where there is great potential for the situation to worsen, and where effective targets can be set.

Case for air pollution as a key area

The largely invisible cocktail of pollutants produced by road traffic and industry includes substances known to be harmful to man.[4] Nitrogen dioxide and sulphur dioxide are respiratory irritants. They are the major constituents of acid rain and exacerbate asthma and chronic lung disease.[5] Airborne particulates, emitted mainly from diesel vehicles and visible in the air as black smoke, are inhaled into the lungs and carry with them acidic gases and volatile organic compounds like benzene, which is a known carcinogen. There is continuing debate about the role of diesel exhaust and benzene in the aetiology of non-occupational lung cancer.[67] Carbon monoxide reduces the oxygen carrying capacity of blood by forming carboxy-haemoglobin. It exacerbates ischaemic heart disease and can precipitate cardiac arrhythmias.[8] Ozone, produced by the effect of sunlight on traffic fumes, causes impaired lung function and, with long term exposure, may cause structural damage to the lungs (Sherwin RP, Richyers V, meeting of the Air and Waste Management Association, Los Angeles, March 1990). There is also some evidence that urban air pollution is responsible for an increase in the prevalence and severity of asthma.[9]

Whether and to what extent these pollutants damage health remains controversial. But the factors responsible for air pollution are increasing. Department of Transport figures predict that the number of cars will double from 23 million to 56 million by 2025, and the growth of the world's population will present ever growing demands on industry and energy production. Unless action is taken air pollution and its effects on health will also increase.

Case against

It could be argued that enormous improvements have already been made in the quality of urban air since the London fog of 1952 in which 4000 people died. And not everyone agrees that modern air pollution is harmful. Laboratory studies on individual pollutants cannot accurately reflect the real situation of a cocktail of pollutants interacting with one another, and population studies are bedevilled by the difficulty of finding unaffected control groups. Cleaning up industry and developing cleaner technology is also likely to be costly, at least in the short term. Other cheaper and more certain routes to a healthy population may seem more attractive priorities.

The targets

The government's targets for reducing air pollution are based on European Community directives (box). These are negotiated for each country and Britain has managed, by a process of stalling and special pleading, to commit itself to less stringent reductions than other European countries with comparable economies. Germany, Denmark, Italy, and France, for example, are committed to a 40% reduction in the production of nitrogen oxides from existing large combustion plants by 1998. Britain's target is 30%. Britain also

143

Government's suggested targets for air pollution

Emissions of nitrogen oxides contribute to acid rain and to photochemical oxidants. The principal sources are large combustion plants such as power stations and vehicles. Action is in hand to reduce emissions from both these sources.

Under certain weather conditions the WHO guideline for peak ozone concentration in air is occasionally exceeded in parts of southern England. Solving this problem will require national and international action to reduce emissions of nitrogen oxides and of volatile organic compounds, which are the precursors of ozone.

- On a 1980 baseline, reduce emissions of nitrogen oxides from existing large combustion plants by 30% by 1988
- Reduce concentrations of nitrogen oxides in urban air on a 1990 baseline by at least 50% by 2000
- By 2000 effective national and supranational controls should be in place to ensure that air quality meets the WHO guideline for peak ozone concentration

negotiated a smaller reduction in production of sulphur dioxide than other European Community countries on the grounds that its coal contains high levels of sulphur. But Britain now imports much of its coal from abroad. What is achievable by comparable economies in Europe and North America should be achievable in Britain. The government should commit itself to a 40% reduction in production of nitrogen oxides from large combustion plants by 1998 and a 70% reduction in production of sulphur dioxide by 2003.

Air quality

Such broad percentage reductions bear little relation to the protection of health at a local level. For this the government should turn to the World Health Organisation's guidelines on air quality. Formulated in 1987 at a meeting of 130 experts from Europe and North America, these give the safe maximum one hour, eight hour, daily, or annual concentrations for various pollutants based on available scientific evidence.[10] They are the best estimates we have of what is necessary to prevent damage to health. WHO guidelines on

World Health Organisation's air quality guidelines and when exceeded in Britain according to Warren Springs Laboratory, the government's monitoring agency

	WHO air quality guideline	When exceeded
Nitrogen dioxide:		
1 h mean	$400 \, \mu g/m^3$	Likely to be exceeded at busy
24 h mean	$150 \, \mu g/m^3$	roadsides
Ozone:		
1 h mean	$150\text{-}200 \, \mu g/m^3$	Exceeded several times during
8 h mean	$100\text{-}120 \, \mu g/m^3$	hot summer of 1989; a site in Devon reached $270 \, \mu g/m^3$
Sulphur dioxide:		
10 min mean	$500 \, \mu g/m^3$	1 h mean regularly exceeded
1 h mean	$350 \, \mu g/m^3$	in London and probably throughout Britain
Airborne particulates:		
24 h mean (in presence of $\geqslant 125 \, \mu g/m^3$ sulphur dioxide)	$125 \, \mu g/m^3$ black smoke or $120 \, \mu g/m^3$ total suspended particulates	Exceeded in 34 sites in 1985-6, mainly due to domestic burning of coal
Carbon monoxide: (To prevent carboxyhaemoglobin concentrations $>2 \cdot 5\text{-}3 \cdot 0\%$ in non-smokers)		
Up to 15 min	$100 \, \mu g/m^3$	At 1 site in London exceeded on
30 min	$60 \, \mu g/m^3$	24 days during winter of 1988. Highest reading almost double the guideline concentration
Benzene	Because benzene is a known carcinogen WHO is unable to recommend a safe level	

safe peak concentrations of all the main air pollutants are regularly exceeded in Britain (table).[11]

Japan, Switzerland, the Netherlands, and the United States all have mandatory air quality standards which are in some cases more stringent than the WHO guidelines. By contrast, the European Community directives are less stringent and do not include any legislation on peak ozone or carbon monoxide concentration. The government's target of adopting the WHO guidelines on peak ozone concentration by 2000 is a step in the right direction. By the same year it should also adopt the WHO guidelines for nitrogen dioxide, sulphur dioxide, carbon monoxide, and airborne particulates.

The green paper does not mention the main greenhouse gas carbon dioxide. The government is already committed to stabilising emissions at 1990 levels by 2005. This target has been described as "feeble" by the environmental group Friends of the Earth. Targets elsewhere in Europe are more ambitious. Germany, for example, plans to cut

145

emissions of carbon dioxide by up to 30% over the same period. The second world climate conference in Geneva last year concluded that cuts of 20% were both technically feasible and cost effective for industrialised countries. The British government should commit itself to a 20% reduction in emissions of carbon dioxide by 2005.

Achieving the targets

The way in which governments choose to tackle environmental pollution depends greatly on the prevailing political ethos. In America there is new interest in the idea of harnessing economic forces to the environmental bandwagon. There is talk of taxation systems that would direct the social and environmental costs of a product back to the producer and pollution tokens that could be traded like stock dividends. Speaking to commercialists in their own language might quickly bring them to a more healthy respect for their environment.

But wedded as it is to Europe, Britain is more likely to take as its model Brussels, with its love of legislative limits, than America, with its unrestrained market forces. In this case the government will need a coherent plan of action incorporating both national and local regulation. Industry and transport should be given separate quotas for pollutants, and targets should be challenging but potentially achievable. If, like much of current European Community and British legislation on air pollution, they are based on what can be achieved with current technology rather than on what is considered necessary to prevent damage to health, they will simply encourage complacency. Legislation should be used to force the pace of industry. The government should set the limits and then determine policy, not the other way round.

Targets for industry

Existing power stations should be fitted with pollution control devices to reduce sulphur dioxide emissons. Tough controls are needed to reduce solvent emissions from paint and print manufacturers. This is an expanding industry and is an important source of volatile organic compounds, which interact with nitrogen dioxide to produce ozone. Companies which introduce cleaner and energy efficient technology should receive financial rewards and those that continue to pollute the atmosphere should be penalised. Britain needs an environmental agency with real power to take action. The United States Environmental Protection Agency, for example, can ban all new development in an area that fails to meet the air quality standards, and in the Netherlands companies can be forced to cut production if pollution exceeds acceptable levels.

Road transport

The area with most scope for reducing air pollution is road transport. It is responsible for the emission of a fifth of carbon dioxide in air, a third of airborne particulates and volatile organic compounds, half of nitrogen oxides, and almost all the carbon monoxide. Catalytic converters will greatly reduce the emission from petrol engines of nitrogen and sulphur dioxides, and filters fitted to diesel engines will reduce particulate and gaseous emissions. Britain has committed itself to existing European Community legislation enforcing the fitting of catalytic converters to all new cars by January 1993 as well as tighter standards on particulate and gaseous emissions for all new trucks and buses by 1996. Similar controls for trucks and buses will be in force two years earlier in the United States, and since European manufacturers are already gearing themselves up for this in order not to lose the American market the European standard could be brought forward to 1994. Friends of the Earth are now campaigning for filters to be fitted to all existing trucks and buses.

Improvements in car design, and the shift from petrol to diesel engines, which emit fewer volatile organic compounds and less carbon monoxide, will reduce air pollution, as will the development of lower sulphur fuels. The amount of benzene and other volatile hydrocarbons escaping into the air will be reduced by the introduction of carbon canisters to absorb fuel vapour at petrol stations.

But technological fixes have their limits. Introducing catalytic converters will result in an initial downturn in emissions of oxides of nitrogen, but the growth in the volume of traffic will soon overcome this. Emissions of exhaust fumes will be on the increase again by the beginning of the next century.[12] For the same reason, carbon dioxide emissions will nearly double by 2020 despite stabilisation of industrial and domestic emissions. Long term reductions in air pollution will be achieved only if traffic is restrained.

The Public Health Alliance has produced a detailed examination of transport policies that would promote health and reduce the burden of road traffic.[13] These include improved public transport systems and town planning; a shift away from factors that encourage people to buy and use cars such as out of town shopping and recreation facilities; changes in the tax system, which currently favours car users; and the

147

transfer of freight from road to rail. Such measures would also reduce road accident deaths and noise pollution and create a more humane urban environment.

Problems

There are obvious obstacles and disincentives to achieving these targets. Traffic restraint will be politically unpopular. The private car symbolises personal freedom and social status, and despite evidence that it has a negative influence on the quality of community life it is often used as a measure of standard of living. Powerful lobbies for the motor industry make sure that these images are maintained.

The improvements in terms of individual health are likely to be small and difficult to measure, especially when dealing with such multifactorial conditions as asthma, chronic bronchitis, and ischaemic heart disease. This absence of neatly quantifiable cause and effect could prove an additional disincentive. Progress will have to be monitored in terms of concentrations of the pollutants in the environment.

Whether or not the economic cost is an obstacle depends on the political will of the government and therefore to some extent on the priorities of the electorate. But because reducing air pollution goes hand in hand with efficient use of energy, in the long term there will be benefits for the economy as well as the nation's health.

1 Secretary of State for Health. *The health of the nation*. London: HMSO, 1991. (Cm 1523.)
2 Wheeler D. Risk assessment and the public perception of water quality. In: *Engineering for health*. London: Institution of Water and Environmental Management, 1990.
3 Reid DD. Air pollution as a cause of chronic bronchitis. *Proceedings of the Royal Society of Medicine* 1964;**57**:965.
4 Read RC, Green M. Internal combustion and health. *BMJ* 1990;**300**:761-2.
5 Ostro BD, Lipsett MJ, Wiener MB, Selner JC. Asthmatic responses to airborne acid aerosols. *Am J Public Health* 1991;**81**:694-702.
6 Steenland K. Lung cancer and diesel exhaust: a review. *Am J Ind Med* 1986;**10**:177-89.
7 International Agency for Research on Cancer. *Diesel and gasoline engine exhausts and some nitroarenes*. Lyons: IARC, 1989. (IARC monographs on the evaluation of carcinogenic risks to humans vol 46.)
8 Alfred EN, Bleeker ER, Chaitman BR, Dahms TE, Gottlieb SO. Short term effects of carbon monoxide exposure on the exercise performance of subjects with coronary artery disease. *N Engl J Med* 1989;**321**:1426-32.
9 Read C. *Air pollution and child health*. London: Greenpeace, 1990.
10 World Health Organisation. *Air quality guidelines for Europe*. Copenhagen: WHO, 1987.
11 Friends of the Earth. *Air quality briefing sheet*. London: Friends of the Earth, 1990.
12 Fergusson M, Holman C, Barrett M. *Atmospheric emissions from the use of transport in the United Kingdom. Vol 1. The estimate of current and future emissions*. London: Worldwide Fund for Nature, Earth Resources Research, 1989.
13 Transport and Health Study Group. Health on the move: a policy statement. Birmingham: Public Health Alliance, 1991.

Housing

STELLA LOWRY

Florence Nightingale understood that "the connection between health and the dwellings of the population is one of the most important that exists," and recent reviews have emphasised that poor housing is still a major threat to public health.[1] No attempt to improve the health of the nation should ignore the benefits of tackling some of our housing problems, but the temptations to do so are great. Although the government acknowledges the importance of housing in its green paper, it fails to set any definite targets (box).[2]

Housing affects health, but in ways that are hard to untangle. The effects of housing may be compounded by those of poverty, age, pre-existing illness, and personal behaviour. Children living in a damp home may have respiratory problems, but if their parents smoke is it fair to blame the housing conditions for the illness? Living in a high rise block may be unhealthy for a single mother of three but ideal for a young working couple with no dependents. An old person living in cold conditions is at increased risk of illness, but this may be the result of unwillingness to turn on a heater, inability to remember how to do it, insufficient money to pay the fuel bills, or a host of other factors rather than a specific defect in the housing.

Studies of housing and health can rarely show a cause and effect relation. Evidence accumulates slowly and usually applies to populations rather than individuals. It is seldom possible to alter a variable and assess the response. But enough is known about the main associations between housing conditions and health to enable some specific targets to be set. These are best phrased in terms of housing targets rather than health targets, and their effects should be monitored in the same way. Many will not show obvious health effects

> ## Green paper focus on housing conditions and homelessness
>
> The overall objective of the government's housing policy is to ensure that decent housing is within reach of all families. Housing policy and programmes continue to give priority to renovation of the housing stock and to securing housing for those who could not otherwise afford decent housing.
>
> Tackling homelessness is a particular priority, not least because of the damage it can cause to people's physical and mental health and wellbeing. Two categories are of particular concern: firstly, single people sleeping rough in the streets (3000-5000), particularly in London, and, secondly, families (11 000) living in bed and breakfast accommodation. Special measures have been introduced to help those sleeping rough in London and to reduce the need for local authorities to use bed and breakfast accommodation; over two years these are expected to provide 16 000 additional family lettings and over 3000 extra places in permanent housing and hostels.

for years, and if they are introduced on too small a scale their potential benefits for improving the health of the population may be missed.

Temperature and humidity

Some of the strongest evidence for effects of housing conditions on health concerns the effects of cold damp homes.[34] The strength of the evidence has been recognised in court rulings.[5] Yet no specific standards for temperature or indoor humidity are included in the building regulations.

Ideally all homes should be capable of being heated to 21°C, the winter room temperature recommended by the British Geriatrics Society. The people who are most vulnerable to the effects of cold and damp often live in poor quality homes that are hard to heat, and these groups are often those who can least afford hefty fuel bills. The poor spend about twice as much, as a percentage of their income, on heating as the rich.[6] It is unreasonable to expect people to spend more than 10% of their household income on heating.

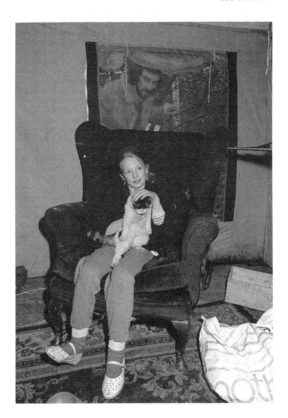

Without increased availability of adequate socially rented housing more families may be forced to live in tents

Specifying that houses should be capable of being heated to 21°C by spending not more than 10% of the average household income on fuel would, in the long term, encourage the building of new homes of high structural quality and the proper repair of existing buildings, with obvious benefits to the nation's housing stock and the world's reserves of fossil fuel. In the short term any excess money needed to meet the heating target for a dwelling should be provided by social payments based on individual needs assessments.

Indoor air quality

Many of the contaminants of indoor air are generated by the occupants of a building. Incorrect use of heating and cooking equipment can increase the content of carbon dioxide, carbon monoxide, and nitrogen dioxide in a home. Smoking also causes considerable contamination of indoor air. It is unrealistic to set targets for those aspects of indoor air quality that rely so heavily on personal behaviour.

Some pollutants are, however, amenable to action. The suggested targets for temperature would also reduce the number of damp homes and have beneficial effects on the levels of house dust mite antigen and fungal spores in indoor air. Both are known to be important causes of respiratory disease, especially in children.[7][8]

Radon is the indoor air pollutant most amenable to target setting. It accounts for nearly half of the average annual exposure to radiation in Britain. The National Radiological Protection Board estimates that the exposure to the national average domestic concentration (20 Bq/m^3) carries a 0·3% lifetime risk of developing lung cancer.[9] The board recommends that radon concentrations in new homes should be as low as possible and certainly not greater than 200 Bq/m^3. It also advises that action should be taken in existing dwellings if the average concentration of radon is above 200 Bq/m^3, and this would probably involve more than 75 000 homes. There is no correlation, however, between the distribution of deaths from lung cancer and domestic exposure to radon. It therefore seems unreasonable to set targets for existing dwellings, but because it makes sense to reduce people's total exposure to radiation all new houses should meet the board's guidelines.

Accidents at home

Each year 5500 fatal and over 3 million non-fatal accidents occur in British homes. Domestic accidents in England and Wales cost the health service £300 million a year. It is difficult to legislate to prevent many of these because individual behaviour is such a large factor in many accidents and personal freedom is important. Most progress will be made by better public education linked with specific personal advice given opportunistically by health workers and other professionals.

An exception to this general principle is the use of architectural glass in houses. Over 400 000 people are injured by domestic glazing each year. The current regulations and terminology are inadequate and confusing.[10] All architectural glass used in new domestic buildings should be toughened glass, which automatically meets class A requirements of British Standard 6202.

Homelessness

In 1989, 162 264 people were accepted as being officially homeless in Britain. The housing charity Shelter estimates that there are two million single homeless people. About 6000 people sleep rough on British streets each night. There are an estimated 1·2 million "hidden homeless" living in overcrowded or unfit conditions but not appearing in the official statistics. The health consequences of homelessness are well documented.[11-13]

Despite recent attempts by the government to increase the number of hostel places available for homeless people the only real solution to these problems is a reversal of attitudes to public sector building and a huge expansion in the number of homes available at low rents. Shelter estimates that about two million families will need a socially rented home in the next five years, and if current trends persist there is likely to be a shortfall of about 600 000 homes.[14] At least 100 000 new homes for rent will be needed each year for the next five years to tackle this crisis.

In conclusion, targets can be set to improve housing in Britain. My suggestions are that:

All homes should be capable of being heated to 21°C by spending not more than 10% of the average household income (any excess needed should be provided from social funds); new houses should be built to ensure that average indoor concentrations of radon do not exceed 200 Bq/m³; all architectural glass used in new homes should be toughened glass meeting British Standard 6202; and public sector building should be increased to provide 100 000 new homes to rent each year for the next five years.

1 Lowry S. *Housing and health.* London: British Medical Journal, 1991.
2 Secretary of State for Health. *The health of the nation.* London: HMSO, 1991. (Cm 1523.)
3 Martin CJ, Platt SD, Hunt SM. Housing conditions and ill health. *BMJ* 1987;**294**:1125-7.
4 Platt SD, Martin CJ, Hunt SM, Lewis CW. Damp housing, mould growth, and symptomatic health state. *BMJ* 1989;**298**:1673-8.
5 Dyer C. Damages for bad housing aggravating asthma. *BMJ* 1990;**301**:781.
6 Boardman B. *Defining affordable warmth.* Warwick: Legal Research Institute, University of Warwick, 1987. (Unhealthy housing: prevention and remedies.)
7 Burr ML, Mullins J, Merrett TG, Stott NCH. Indoor moulds and asthma. *J R Soc Health* 1988;**108**:99-101.
8 Burr ML, Neale E, Dean BV, Verrier-Jones ER. Effect of a change to mite free bedding on children with mite-sensitive asthma: a controlled trial. *Thorax* 1980;**35**:513-4.
9 O'Riordan MC. *Human exposure to radon in homes. Recommendations for the practical application of the Board's statement.* Chilton: National Radiological Protection Board, 1990.
10 Lowry S. *Housing and health.* London: British Medical Journal, 1991:59-66.
11 Conway J, ed. *Prescription for poor health. The crisis for homeless families.* London: London Food Commission, Maternity Alliance, SHAC, Shelter, 1988.
12 Ramsden SS, Baur S, El Kabir DJ. Tuberculosis among the central London single homeless. *J R Coll Physicians Lond* 1988;**22**:16-7.
13 Health Visitors' Association and General Medical Services Committee. *Homeless families and their health.* London: British Medical Association, 1989.
14 Foster S, Burrows L. *Urgent need for homes.* London: Shelter, 1991.

The role of exercise

HENRY J DARGIE, S GRANT

Exercise can take many forms and, at least until now, has been most commonly associated with the prevention of coronary heart disease. But with the accumulating evidence for preventive and therapeutic benefit in many other conditions, exercise is emerging as a key element in most national health promotion recommendations and strategies.[1-5] This is hardly surprising as the ability to exercise is intrinsic to most aspects of human life and simple physical training can enable even the most unfit people and those limited by chronic illness to carry out the basic activities of modern sedentary life more efficiently and comfortably.[6]

Exercise as a key area

The importance of coronary artery disease in Western society is not sufficient to justify including exercise as a key area. It must also be possible to conclude that exercise can favourably influence the occurrence or natural course of coronary heart disease[7] and other conditions.

Coronary heart disease

That exercise might be protective in coronary heart disease is biologically plausible even if the scientific evidence is not universally accepted.[8 9] Exercise could exert benefits by its effects on the main coronary risk factors.[10 11] Thus aerobic exercise reduces blood pressure,[12] increases high density lipoprotein concentration,[13] facilitates stopping smoking,[14] and reduces obesity.[15] Recent evidence, however, suggests that it may act on the acute phase of coronary heart disease, possibly on the coagulation mechanism or even arrhythmia.[16 17]

Many epidemiological studies have investigated the relation between work and leisure time exercise and coronary heart disease[18-21]; the evidence strongly favours the view that regular aerobic exercise of moderate intensity has a protective effect, and the benefit probably increases with the intensity of exercise. Morris, one of the earliest proponents of the protective effects of exercise, recently calculated that regular dynamic exercise of moderate intensity reduced the incidence of coronary events and mortality from coronary heart disease by up to 50%.[17]

Meta-analyses of controlled studies of exercise training after myocardial infarction suggest a reduction of about 25% in recurrent infarction and sudden death from heart failure.[22] As most of those who die of coronary heart disease are already known to have this or other vascular disease,[23] the impressive contribution of exercise in secondary prevention should not be underestimated.

Osteoporosis

Hip fractures, which are a common manifestation of osteoporosis, are an important cause of morbidity, and patients often require expensive institutional care. In 1985 in England 37 600 people fractured a hip, and one in four women reaching the age of 90 can be expected to have a hip fracture.[24]

Bone density is greater in athletes than in age matched normal sedentary people.[25] Exercise programmes in postmenopausal women can also increase bone density and reverse the normal postmenopausal bone loss seen in women who do not exercise. The risk of hip fracture is substantially reduced in those who exercise regularly. Moreover, in elderly people exercise reduces the likelihood of falling.[26] It is estimated that regular exercise would reduce the risk of fracture by as much as a half, thereby preventing some 20 000 hip fractures each year.[24]

Several strategies could help reduce the cost of health care in elderly people and among these, certainly for hip fracture, exercise is arguably the most important. The potential for exercise in facilitating greater self care remains to be explored more fully.

Obesity

Obesity is endemic in modern society and is much more important than its modest contribution to the prevalence of coronary heart disease would suggest. Although changes in body composition with exercise are variable, it is generally accepted that total body mass and fat weight are reduced. Fat free weight remains constant or may increase slightly. Energy reduced diets, by contrast, lower both fat weight and fat free weight. When energy reduced diets are combined with exercise, the fat free weight loss is considerably less compared with programmes using only diet.[27] Exercise has a complementary role in encouraging energy expenditure as well as strengthening the resolve to lose weight by promoting greater self esteem and enhanced morale.[28]

The physiological benefits associated with training are relatively easily attainable and could be valuable in numerous human diseases that impair human performance. Patients who might benefit include those with chronic renal failure receiving regular dialysis (who have considerably impaired physical ability),[29] depression,[30] respiratory disease,[31] and late onset diabetes.[1]

The case against

Some would argue that there is no conclusive evidence from controlled trials that regular exercise reduces the number of deaths from coronary heart disease or substantially prolongs life. To demand such proof is to miss the main point about exercise, which is that it is valuable for the numerous other health benefits it confers and as a catalyst in the adoption of a healthier lifestyle.

Regular exercise has some disadvantages, which include expense— equipment, use of leisure centres, and sports complexes are not necessarily cheap—and personal injury—although exercise might prevent hip fractures in elderly people, stress fractures and joint problems associated with specific sports are well recognised but poorly catered for by the embryonic specialty of sports medicine. Occasional deaths during running events and other sporting activities underline the point that intense exercise can be dangerous, especially in those with unsuspected underlying heart disease.[32] Paradoxically, appropriate exercise training can increase exercise capacity and reduce symptoms in patients with angina[33] and even with heart failure.[34]

The government has suggested several diseases where action could be taken to improve the nation's health.[5] Most human disease is multifactorial in origin, and a good example of that is coronary heart disease. But even where a single, well defined aetiological agent is identified, such as HIV in AIDS, many other factors are involved. Thus, even in apparently well defined diseases "non-specific" measures to improve the state of an individual's health could be important. Health is not merely the absence of disease, and, while few would care to define it, a sense of wellbeing and fitness should be central to any initiative to promote health. Thus exercise should be a key factor in health promotion because it can provide that feeling of wellbeing not only in those who are well (that is, those without any specific named disease) but in those with illnesses that restrict their performance.[6 29 35]

Targets for exercise

The personal targets for exercise will vary according to the primary desired effect. It is possible to identify a variety of components of exercise—skeletal (muscle, bone, and joints), cardiovascular, and energy balance. It could be argued that the type of exercise should be targeted at the disease process. Thus weight bearing or strength exercises might be best for preventing osteoporosis and hip fracture.[6] Such exercise requires a small increase in energy expenditure.

For preventing coronary heart disease, dynamic exercise such as running, swimming, or cycling is necessary. A significant training effect can be obtained by exercise which raises the heart rate above resting levels by 50% of the heart rate range for 30 minutes at least three times a week.[27]

Several physical activities could be recommended for maintaining

---

Possibility of government targets for exercise

More needs to be known about current participation in physical activity, exercise, and sport and current fitness

A national fitness survey was launched in 1990. This will provide "benchmark" data on fitness, participation, and effectiveness of different types of exercise

The government will examine the survey's findings and in the light of these consider possible targets. Physical activity will then be a prime candidate for inclusion as a key area in the health strategy

---

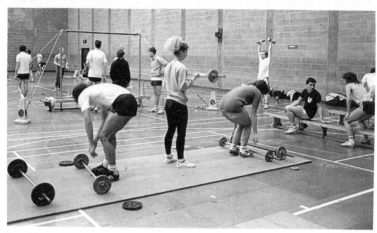

Group fitness programmes can be fun

the energy balance at a desirable level of body fatness or for preventing or treating obesity. These activities would require expending considerable amounts of energy (8 kJ/min) over several hours—for example, by playing golf—and have little effect on the cardiovascular system.[8]

Thus, an exercise programme can be tailored to the needs of the individual but, in general terms, components of each type of exercise can be incorporated into exercise prescriptions. The government, however, has not as yet suggested any targets for physical activity (box).

Strategy for reaching targets

Individual and population strategies should be complementary. Population studies suggest that only a few people take adequate exercise.[36] Adherence to exercise programmes is notoriously poor, with a typical drop out rate from supervised programmes of around 50% in various countries. Further research is needed to establish what determines the amount of exercise people take so that physical activity can be increased.[37] It is unlikely that the promise of a few months extra life would be sufficiently tempting to encourage such a dramatic change of lifestyle. Such promises should be abandoned in favour of a strategy that portrays exercise as being a part of or indeed the catalyst in a lifestyle change that might include several other components, such as stopping smoking, nutritional change, reduction in stress, etc.[38] To do this, exercise must be enjoyable, affordable, and accessible. Health promotion clinics in general practice could identify those who might benefit from an exercise programme.

Home based exercise programmes may be successful, though group fitness sessions at leisure centres or sports clubs can be enjoyable. Education and motivation to improve scores are sound reasons for offering regular fitness assessments. But these would require access to people with appropriate expertise, who would best be located in sports centres where community based exercise programmes could develop.

Participation of the media is essential; there are few campaigns to increase uptake of exercise and these could be increased. Encouraging walking or cycling to work together with providing exercise facilities at work and promoting of exercise and health maintenance during work could help. The establishment of many more cycle tracks and lanes could be the single measure that would be most effective in encouraging an active lifestyle. The importance of schools encouraging regular participation in sport and the adoption of an active lifestyle cannot be overstated.

Problems

A major barrier to greater participation in exercise is the relative paucity of adequate exercise and sporting facilities. This should not be a deterrent to or be a part of the case against exercise being a key area: but it would be pointless to advocate exercise to a population that had inadequate facilities to partake in it. Availability of sports centres, especially in deprived areas, and their expense are key issues. Trained professionals to supervise and advise will be required, and sports medicine facilities might also be needed.

A national fitness survey is necessary to discover the true fitness of the nation and, for England at least, this information will shortly be available. Whether the results of this survey will lead to the establishment of realistic targets and proposals to improve health through regular physical activity remains to be seen. It will cost money and it is to be hoped that the government will provide the resources to establish a coordinated structure for promoting increased physical activity.

1 Royal College of Physicians Medical aspects of exercise: benefits and risks. *J R Coll Physicians Lond* 1991;25:193-6.

2 British Cardiac Society Working Group on Coronary Prevention. Conclusions and recommendations. *Br Heart J* 1987;**57**:188-9.

3 Scottish Home and Health Department and Scottish Health Service Advisory Council. *Prevention of coronary heart disease in Scotland. Report of the working group on prevention and health promotion.* Edinburgh: HMSO, 1990.

4 Scottish Home and Health Department. *Health education in Scotland: a national policy statement.* Edinburgh: SHHD, 1991.

5 Secretary of State for Health. *The health of the nation.* London: HMSO, 1991. (Cm 1523.)

6 Fentem PH, Bassey EJ, Turnbull NB. *The new case for exercise.* London: Health Education Authority, 1988.

7 Shephard RJ. Exercise in coronary heart disease. *Sports Med* 1986;**3**:26-49.

8 Durnin JVGA. *Report submitted to the COMA committee on diet and cardiovascular disease.* London: Department of Health, 1984.

9 Leon AR. The relationship of physical activity to coronary heart disease and life expectancy. *Ann N Y Acad Sci* 1977;**301**:561-78.

10 Cooper KH, Pollock ML, Martin RP, White SR, Linneryd AC, Jackson A. Physical fitness levels *vs* selected coronary risk factors. *JAMA* 1976;**236**: 166-9.

11 Poole GW. Exercise, coronary heart disease and risk factors. A brief report. *Sports Med* 1984;**1**:341-9.

12 Duncan JJ, Farr JE, Upton SJ, Hagan RD, Oglesby ME, Blair SN. The effects of aerobic exercise on plasma catecholamines and blood pressure in patients with mild essential hypertension. *JAMA* 1985;**254**:2609-13.

13 Goldberg L, Elliot DL. The effect of exercise on lipid metabolism in men and women. *Sports Med* 1987;**4**:307-21.

14 Marcus BH, Albrecht AE, Niaura RS, Abrams DB, Thompson PD. Usefulness of physical exercise for maintaining smoking cessation in women. *Am J Cardiol* 1991;**68**:406-7.

15 Bray GA. Exercise and obesity. In: Bouchard C, Shephard RJ, Stephens T, Sutton JR, McPherson BD, eds. *Exercise, fitness and health. A consensus of current knowledge.* Champaign, Illinois: Human Kinetics Books, 1988:497-510.

16 Fentem P, Turnbull NB. Benefits of exercise for heart health: a report on the scientific basis. In: *Exercise heart health: report of a conference organised by the coronary prevention group.* London: Coronary Prevention Group, 1987:110-25.

17 Morris JN, Clayton DG, Everitt MG, Semmence AM, Burgess EH. Exercise in leisure time: coronary attack and death rates. *Br Heart J* 1990;**63**:325-34.

18 Morris HM, Heady JA, Raffle PAB, Roberts GC, Parks JW. Coronary heart disease and physical activity of work. *Lancet* 1953;ii:1053-4.

19 Morris JN, Chave SPW, Adam C, Sirey C, Epstein L, Sheehan DJ. Vigorous exercise in leisure-time and the incidence of coronary heart disease. *Lancet* 1973;i:333-9.

20 Paffenberger RS, Weng AL, Hyde RT. Physical activity as an index of heart attack risk in college alumni. *Am J Epidemiol* 1978;**108**:161-75.

21 Powell KE, Thomson PD, Caspersen CJ, Hendrick JS. Physical activity and the incidence of coronary heart disease. *Annu Rev Public Health* 1987;**8**: 253-87.

22 O'Connor GT, Buring JE, Yusuf S, Goldhaber SZ, Olmstead EM, Paffenberger RS Jr, *et al.* An overview of randomised trials of rehabilitation with exercise after myocardial infarction. *Circulation* 1989;**80**:234-44.

23 Tunstall-Pedoe H, Clayton D, Morris JN, Brigden W, McDonald L. Coronary heart-attacks in East London. *Lancet* 1975;ii:833-8.

24 Law MR, Wald NJ, Meade TW. Strategies for prevention of osteoporosis and hip fracture. *BMJ* 1991;**303**:453-9.

25 Smith EL, Gilgan C. Effects of inactivity and exercise on bone. *Physician and Sports Medicine* 1987;**15**:91-102.

26 Fiatarone MA, Marks EC, Ryan DT, Meredith CN, Lipsitz LA, Evans WJ. High-intensity strength training in nonagenarians: effects on skeletal muscle. *JAMA* 1990;**263**:3029-34.

27 American College of Sports Medicine. The recommended quantity and quality of exercise for developing and maintaining cardiorespiratory and muscular fitness in healthy adults. *Med Sci Sports Exerc* 1990;**22**:265-74.

28 Garfinkel PE, Coscina DV. Discussion: Exercise and obesity. In: Bouchard C, Shephard RJ, Stephens T, Sutton JR, McPherson BD, eds. *Exercise fitness and health. A consensus of current knowledge.* Champaign, Illinois: Human Kinetics Books, 1988:455-66.

29 Goldberg AP, Geltman E, Gavin JR, Carney RM, Hagberg JM, Delmez JA, *et al.* Exercise

training reduces coronary risk and effectively rehabilitates haemodialysis patients. *Nephron* 1986;**42**:311-6.

30 Brown DR. Exercise, fitness and mental health. In: Bouchard C, Shephard RJ, Stephens T, Sutton JR, McPherson BD, eds. *Exercise, fitness and health. A consensus of current knowledge.* Champaign, Illinois: Human Kinetics Books, 1988:607-26.

31 Consensus statement. In: Bouchard C, Shephard RJ, Stephens T, Sutton JR, McPherson BD, eds. *Exercise fitness and health. A consensus of current knowledge.* Champaign, Illinois: Human Kinetics Books: 1988:3-28.

32 Northcote RJ, Ballantyne D. Sudden death and sport. *Sports Med* 1984;**1**: 181-6.

33 Tood IC, Ballantyne D. Antianginal efficacy of exercise training: a comparison with beta blockade. *Br Heart J* 1990;**64**:14-9.

34 Sullivan MJ, Higginbotham MB, Cobb FR. Exercise training in patients with severe left ventricular dysfunction, hemodynamic and metabolic effects. *Circulation* 1988;**78**:506-15.

35 Folkins CH, Wesley ES. Physical fitness training and mental health. *Am Psychol* 1981;**36**: 373-89.

36 Tunstall-Pedoe H, Smith WCS, Crombie IK, Tavendale R. Coronary risk factor and lifestyle variation across Scotland: results from the Scottish Heart Health Study. *Scot Med J* 1989;**34**:556-60.

37 Dishman RK. Exercise adherence: its impact on public health. In: Hermans GPH, Mosterd W. *Proceedings of the XXIV world congress of sports medicine.* Amsterdam: Elsevier Science Publishers, 1990:11-21.

38 Work JA. How healthy are corporate fitness programs? *Physician and Sports Medicine* 1989;**3**:226-37.

Work related disorders

J M HARRINGTON

The consultative document on a strategy for health is described as a new concept for England.[1] It is, and as such should be warmly welcomed. The fact that it is woolly in some places and seriously deficient in others does not detract from its importance as a first step in the right direction. The purpose of the consultation phase is to highlight those deficiencies and sharpen the focus elsewhere. One of the document's deficiencies is the scant attention it gives to occupational health.

Should work related diseases and injuries be a key area?

There are nearly 30 million people of employable age in England and Wales, which, even in these times of high unemployment, means a large number of people at work. Occupational health services of one sort or another are available to about half these people. Most companies employing more than 1000 people have full or part time medical and nursing staff with occupational health qualifications. The underresourced Health and Safety Executive, through its employment medical advisers, attempts to provide some degree of care for the rest.

This working population faces a variety of work-place hazards. The latest figures (for 1988-9) from the Health and Safety Executive indicate that 514 deaths occurred that year (including 167 in the Piper Alpha disaster), with 150 000 people receiving injuries requiring at least three days off work.[2] Though these figures show a slight fall year on year, they are actually a considerable underestimate of reality. For what they are worth they suggest one new case of work related disease eligible for compensation per 4500 employees. The equivalent statistics from Finland are 10 times worse while in Sweden the annual reported rate is one case per 100 employees. This reflects, without doubt, more effective recording in Scandinavia, not better British work practices.[3]

If the diseases and injuries are extended beyond "work caused" to "work related" what meagre evidence is available suggests that for mortality the work relatedness varies from 12% for cancer to 25% for cardiovascular diseases[4]—equivalent to 1800 premature deaths a year among men of employable age.

Diseases and injuries caused by work are all theoretically preventable. Indeed the ability to prevent rests largely with the employers and government. As the first medical inspector of factories, Sir Thomas Legge (1863-1932), said: "Unless and until the employer has done everything—and everything means a good deal—the workman can do next to nothing to protect himself, although he is naturally willing to do his share."[5] Such a division of responsibility for health and safety at work is enshrined in the Health and Safety at Work Act 1974.

Prevention of ill health is a cornerstone of occupational health practice. The Secretary of State for Health considers that specific areas deserving special attention include maintaining good health, preventing ill health, rehabilitating people to good health, and supporting disabled people. These are the raison d'être for occupational health services. Such services, staffed by qualified practitioners, thus provide the only logical site for preventing work related disease or

---

Occupational health in the strategy document

The green paper recognises that industry and commerce have responsibilities for improving health and that there is scope for investing in the health of the workforce by:

• Promoting healthy living, ensuring that catering services offer healthy food, and providing exercise facilities

• Offering employees the chance to participate in workplace health initiatives

Nevertheless, no specific role for occupational health professionals is identified either separately or in meeting targets in other key areas

---

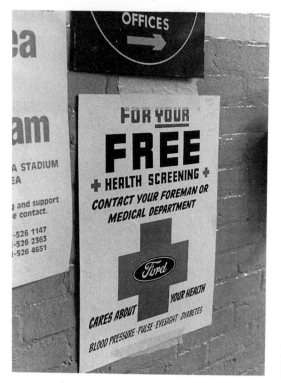

The workplace offers
ideal opportunities for
health promotion

injury; they also provide a crucial location for general health
education and targeted health promotion. The regular opportunities
that occupational health services provide for doctors and nurses to
influence workplace exposures and alter lifestyles that are hazardous
to health could be argued to be unparalleled elsewhere in the health
services. Indeed, given that these services are paid for by employers,
the secretary of state is missing an opportunity to use a "free" health
service.

The problem of responsibility for leading preventive strategies is
bedevilled by the two extreme claims "It's up to individuals" and "It's
all up to government." The consultative document fails to provide a
viable solution, partly because the paper misguidedly concentrates on
the NHS and the Department of Health largely to the exclusion of the
rest. Even if one did espouse such a restricted view, it should be
remembered that the NHS is now the country's largest employer and

has only belatedly woken up to its own health and safety responsibilities for its own enormous workforce.[6]

The case against

The health care of employed people has never been a direct responsibility of the NHS. Since 1947 what government interest has been shown has been considered the responsibility of the Department of Employment and its predecessors. This has, over the years, allowed other government departments—notably health and social security—to abrogate any concern under the guise of not confusing ministerial responsibility.

Such an approach is no longer tenable. Lip service is paid in the consultative document to the need for interdepartmental cooperation and shared responsibilities. However, the issues—and the toll in human suffering from work related disorders—are too important to be left to one department and too central to the strategy for health to be left uncoordinated by central government. The "strong leadership and adequate coordination" advocated for accident prevention in general[7] applies equally to work related injuries and disease. The case against designating work related diseases and injuries as a key area is not merit. It is negligence in interdepartmental cooperation, poverty of resources, and ignorance by the Department of Health that such vital preventive measures can be tackled now by using free health care resources which already exist in many companies but are historically out with the NHS. Occupational health practitioners and their services must feel some ownership of the Waldegrave goals or these goals are further off and less attainable than they would be otherwise.

The key areas

The key areas listed in the document are, with few exceptions, key areas for occupational health practice. Coronary artery disease, though mainly a lifestyle disease, also has work related factors ranging from chemical exposures which cause or exacerbate the disease to stress related influences from the occupations. Olsen and Kristensen recently postulated that 16% of premature deaths from cardiovascular disease in Denmark could be avoided by workplace intervention.[8] On top of that, the occupational health services can, and do, actively participate in preventive initiatives such as Look After Your Heart.

165

Indeed the workplace has been shown to provide an ideal setting for such health promotion.

Workplace exposures cause 3-6% of all cancers and contribute to the development of cancer in a similar percentage.[9] This may be a fairly small fraction compared with smoking or diet, for example, but all the workplace agents can be controlled or eliminated much more readily than can lifestyle factors. For some tumours, such as lung and bladder, it is estimated that the workplace factors may cause up to 40% of these tumours in manual workers aged 20 years or over in mining, agriculture, and broadly defined industry.[10] Thus to concentrate on breast and cervical cancer, which the public perceives as important,[11] ducks the central issues of how to cope with the other, perhaps commoner, tumours; how to tackle cigarette smoking; and how to aid the control of workplace related cancers.

Accidents at work cause injury and the rates are not improving appreciably.[12] The question of accident prevention in general has been dealt with elsewhere in this series.[7] The arguments and issues raised there apply equally well to workplace injuries.

Asthma is of growing concern to public health specialists as it seems to be increasing in both children and adults. Workplace aetiological factors are becoming increasingly recognised and, of late, more reliable statistics are becoming available through the new surveillance scheme.[13] Even so, the Faculty of Occupational Medicine of the Royal College of Physicians of London believes that the estimated 500 cases a year may be an underestimate. Its working party, which is contributing to the Faculty of Public Health Medicine's second report on United Kingdom levels of health (due to be published in mid-1992), suggests a figure nearer 1500 cases would be closer to the truth.

Space does not allow an opportunity to discuss other important disease groupings, such as the 60 000 cases of industrial dermatitis each year. But, for the rest of the key areas such as lifestyle influences, maternal and child health, and rehabilitation occupational health professionals have a part to play in that they care for employed people who will include the pregnant and the disabled. So far as environmental quality is concerned, some of the problem here lies with the industries that pollute. Their occupational health advisers have for some considerable time been an integral part of the environmental control strategies operated by the larger and more enlightened industries. For many of these doctors, environmental health is now of central and increasing importance in their daily work.

Strategies for reaching targets

Others will comment in greater detail, and with greater expertise, on the validity of the government's targets. Some could be stronger. For example, one proposed target from the Faculty of Occupational Medicine working party is for total smoking bans in all enclosed workplaces by the year 2000. For other key areas it should be clear that a vital strategy in setting targets and reaching them is the active participation of workplace based health services and the recognition of the value of such services and their practitioners in the overall scheme of things.

If government departments are going to work together in a co-ordinated way to achieve the green paper's objectives then occupational health has an important role. European legislation is likely to press for increased emphasis on occupational health. Active government support of occupational health services in Britain (as proposed by the House of Lords Select Committee on Science and Technology 1983) could ensure these services are developed so that they can make a significant contribution to health promotion. Such action could also influence the European approach to occupational health screening services, which may otherwise focus on procedures of doubtful benefit. It is therefore timely (if somewhat belated) to introduce into the government's strategy on health a scheme for improving occupational health services for all employees. This need not be expensive as the costs are borne by employers. Government initatives on occupational health are long overdue and this is its opportunity to act.

Problems in achieving targets

The consultative document has been criticised for identifying key areas and setting targets only where data exist on the size of the problem. For occupational health, a major difficulty is the paucity of good quality databases on the size of the work related health problem. The Health and Safety Executive has started to tackle the issue but the Reporting of Injuries, Diseases, and Dangerous Occurrence Regulations has been unevenly successful.[14] For diseases the regulations are a failure. The specific new initiatives for respiratory disease surveillance[13] and now others for urothelial tumours and haematological disorders should gather more accurate information, but as yet we have not shown the same enthusiasm or initiative as the United States Public Health Service in attempting to tackle the serious deficiencies

167

in occupational health and safety surveillance,[15] and in identifying occupational "sentinel health" events.[16] Without this information we do not know the size of the problem, but it seems largely based on known underestimates. Its contribution to the ill health of the nation is considerable on present statistics. Perhaps if and when we have a better estimate, the resources might be made available to tackle a sizable portion of the problem at the heart of the consultative document: the need to improve the health of the nation.

Conclusions

Improving the health of the nation includes the health of employed people—indeed it could be argued that as they are the money earners, their health has particular importance. The consultative document pays little attention to occupational health practice. Yet it is at the workplace, with thousands of qualified professionals serving millions of employees, that special attention could be paid to health promotion in general as well as attacking the unacceptable level of work related disease and injury which weakens the economic and physical health of the country. The overall goals in the Department of Health's proposals are ideally suited to action from these occupational health practitioners. Their skills and their opportunity for intervention makes them essential, perhaps unique, players in the game plan. The fact that the document largely ignores them and the opportunity they provide to influence the nation's health is a serious omission requiring rectification.

1 Secretary of State for Health. *The health of the nation.* London: HMSO, 1991. (Cm 1523.)
2 Health and Safety Executive. *Health and Safety statistics 1988/89.* London: HMSO, 1990. (Employment gazette 98: occasional supplement No 1.)
3 Schilling RSF. Health protection and prevention at work. *Br J Ind Med* 1989;**46**:683-8.
4 Fox AJ, Adelstein AM. Occupational mortality: work or way of life? *J Epidemiol Community Health* 1978;**32**:73-8.
5 Legge TM. In: Henry SA, ed. *Industrial maladies.* London: Oxford University Press, 1934.
6 Harrington JM. The health of the health care workers. The Ernestine Henry Lecture 1990. *J R Coll Physicians Lond* 1990;**24**:189-95.
7 Pless IB. Accident prevention. *BMJ* 1991;**303**:462-4.
8 Olsen O, Kristensen TS. Impact of work environment on cardiovascular diseases in Denmark. *J Epidemiol Community Health* 1991;**45**:4-10.
9 Doll R, Peto R. *The causes of cancer.* Oxford: Oxford University Press, 1981.
10 Harrington JM, Saracci R. Occupational cancer. Raffle PAB, Adams P, Baxter P, Lee WR, eds. *Hunter's diseases of occupation.* 8th ed. Sevenoaks: Hodder and Stoughton (in press).
11 Williams CJ. Cancer. *BMJ* 1991;**303**:576-7.
12 Aw T-C, Harrington JM. Industrial accidents. *BMJ* 1989;**303**:68-9.
13 Meridith SK, Taylor VM, McDonald JC. Occupational respiratory disease in the United Kingdom, 1989: a report to the British Thoracic Society and the Society of Occupational Medicine by the SWORD project group. *Br J Ind Med* 1991;**48**:292-8.

14 Carter JT. There's a lot of it about. *Br J Ind Med* 1991;**48**:289-91.
15 Baker EL, ed. Surveillance in occupational health and safety. *Am J Public Health* 1989;**79** (Suppl 1):64.
16 Mullan RJ, Murthy LI. Occupational sentinel health events: an updated list for physician recognition and public health surveillance. *Am J Ind Med* 1991;**19**:775-99.

Medical genetics

RODNEY HARRIS

Molecular genetics has been responsible for some of the most striking recent developments in medicine. Enormous new opportunities result from the human genome project, with virtually all single gene diseases already mapped to their chromosomal locations. The application of the information gained in this project to clinical practice should be consistent with the aims of medical genetics, which are:

● To ensure the maximum range of options for those at risk of genetic disease by providing accurate diagnosis and screening, empathic genetic counselling, and support

● To prevent genetic disease and unnecessary anxiety by facilitating personal informed choices from among these options

● To aid appropriate clinical management of genetic disease and to identify preventable complications by early and accurate diagnosis.

Below I discuss why medical genetics should be recognised as a key area in the consultations initiated by *The Health of the Nation.*[1]

The case for genetics

Genetic diseases and congenital malformations fulfil all three of the government's criteria for a key area. They are an important cause of premature death and avoidable ill health, there are interventions offering scope for improvement in health, and it is possible to set targets and then to monitor them.

Five per cent of the population will have a genetic disorder by the age of 25. This figure rises to 65% in a lifetime if common diseases with a strong genetic predisposition are included. In addition, 2-3% of couples are at high risk of having handicapped offspring.[2,3] There is also the fear and anxiety generated by recurring genetic disease among relatives at risk of such diseases.

Specific vulnerable groups

The green paper calls for "specific initiatives to address the health needs of particularly vulnerable groups." In medical genetics these groups are pregnant women, neonates, people from ethnic minorities, and those who are found to be positive for genetic defects in population screening programmes.

People with a family history of serious genetic disease are a special group because many common genetic disorders within families can now be avoided. Consistent with the aims of medical genetics, genetic family registers of those at highest risk are the most effective way of assisting relatives of patients with severe genetic disease including hereditary cancer, Duchenne muscular dystrophy, Huntington's chorea, and adult polycystic kidney disease. In the future additional vulnerable groups may be recognised as knowledge grows about the genetic predisposition to common disease (cancer, coronary artery disease, diabetes mellitus, psychosis, etc).

Interventions offering improvements in health

There are well established programmes for preventing genetic and congenital disorders, notably Down's syndrome, neural tube defect, thalassaemia, Tay-Sachs disease, and phenylketonuria. The cost-effectiveness of these programmes has been studied. Screening with ultrasound and of maternal serum α fetoprotein concentrations has contributed to the dramatic reduction in the number of babies born with neural tube defect, while screening based on maternal age and biochemical markers is capable of identifying at least 60% of pregnancies with fetuses affected with Down's syndrome.[4]

New techniques in genetics may facilitate and simplify existing procedures and are often effective in more than one laboratory discipline. Thus the polymerase chain reaction has revolutionised molecular genetics and has applications throughout laboratory medicine. Non-isotopic in situ hybridisation offers greater safety than conventional isotopic methods and has wide applicability in cytogenetics, molecular genetics, and biochemical genetics.

Medical genetics is a dynamic subject in which change occurs very rapidly. Screening for the following conditions will become a public health issue in the near future.

Cancer in families—All cancers are the result of genetic mutations or a failure of gene regulation, often aided and abetted by environmental carcinogens. However, some cancers are inherited in a mendelian fashion. For example, colorectal cancer kills 21 000 people a year— 10 times the figure for cervical cancer—but while bowel screening is technically possible it is not currently practical for the whole adult population at risk. Some colorectal cancers, however, occur in families, including familial adenomatous polyposis and non-adenomatous familial bowel cancer. Such cancers should be preventable by family counselling, regular bowel screening, and appropriate early surgery. These interventions reduce the 10 year mortality from over 80% to 40%.[5] Advances in molecular genetics have made screening more effective and, as a bonus, most relatives could soon be reassured that they are unlikely to carry the cancer gene. This not only gives great relief to the relatives but saves the NHS the expense of regular screening for them and their descendants. There are strong hints that common, sporadic bowel cancer may share similar genetic mutations, and this pattern recurs for many genetic cancers and other disorders. In breast cancer molecular techniques also promise advances in screening in younger women, those for whom mammography is least useful.

Marfan syndrome—The gene for this disorder has now been identified[6] and the basic biochemical defect elucidated. This will provide a new certainty in diagnosis, which is particularly important as the clinical expression of the disease is so variable. The first beneficiaries will be older children and young adults whose close relatives have died of dissecting aneurysm of the aorta. Those who are shown to have the gene will require regular cardiac ultrasonography, prophylactic drugs, and elective heart surgery—thus greatly improving their prognosis. Most relatives will be shown not to be carriers and will require no further screening, which will thus save NHS resources. Relatives will also enjoy considerable relief from anxiety about their own and their children's health.

Fragile X syndrome—Recent molecular genetic advances in the fragile X syndrome[7 8] (carried by perhaps one in 1000 British women) indicate that screening programmes may soon be feasible for carriers of this the most common form of severe inherited mental retardation.

Premature coronary artery disease—One in every 500 of the white population is a carrier of familial hypercholesterolaemia, and all carriers are liable to premature death due to coronary occlusion. Screening and prevention are now possible, but relatives at high risk need to be identified at an early age if prevention is to be effective.

172

An important limiting factor is the need for input from clinical geneticists; at present there are too few to deal with such large numbers of families.

Intersector advantages

Medical genetics depends on multidisciplinary cooperation in the NHS and the community. It has strong advantages in many health sectors because prevention of genetic disease by health service initiatives reduces chronic disability and results in savings which are at their maximum in the community and social services. However, such savings are not always easy to quantify in accountancy terms and tend to be overlooked.

Identifying and monitoring targets

Targets must be identified which are consistent with the fundamental principles of medical genetics, which were outlined at the beginning of the article. The Department of Health anticipated the need for evaluation and funded a four year special medical development to assess the value of molecular genetics in clinical genetics. This showed that genetic services were both cheap and effective, even with the limited procedures then available.[9] Now, specifically to evaluate the management and prevention of genetic disorders by many specialties, the department has commissioned the Royal College of Physicians of London to set up a confidential enquiry into the quality of counselling for genetic disorders. The inquiry will review clinical records of marker disorders (cystic fibrosis, Down's syndrome, familial polyposis, haemophilia, multiple endocrine neoplasia type 2, neural tube defect, and thalassaemia). The targets in each case will be 100% of clinical records having documented evidence of appropriate counselling, of relevant genetic services being offered, and of follow up, especially where potentially preventable late onset disorders are concerned.

The case against

Genetic disorders have, in the past, been regarded as rare and untreatable. There are also reservations about termination of pregnancy, which has erroneously been perceived as the only preventive measure available. Now new genetic screening procedures for familial cancers and other adult onset genetic disease offer different approaches. Reservations about prenatal diagnosis have also been mitigated by rapid technical advances bringing much earlier and more precise diagnosis.[10] Prenatal diagnosis in most cases gives normal results providing enormous relief from anxiety. Indeed, in these situations women are encouraged to begin and to continue pregnancies that might otherwise have been terminated. Medical genetics emphasises the importance of fully informed free choice in reproduction and of the confidentiality of genetic information. This is not only consistent with the ethical importance of recognising the autonomy of the individual but experience shows that it in no way impedes effectiveness because most of those at risk of having offspring with serious handicapping disorders will choose prenatal diagnosis if it is available and if they are given all the relevant information.

There is now overwhelming evidence of general public support for the use of medical genetic advances, as was evident during the proceedings of the Embryo Research Bill. Nevertheless, the unique value of human life must continue to be emphasised, with thoughtfulness and restraint being exercised in all such research. Support for medical genetics is particularly consistent and articulate from lay organisations such as the Genetic Interest Group, which represents more than 60 medical genetic charities.

Need for better education

The generally poor teaching of genetics to medical students and the sometimes doubtful clinical relevance of what they have been taught[11] is a potential barrier at present to the effective involvement of doctors in genetic services. The Royal College of Physicians has also surveyed postgraduate education in genetics (A W Johnston, personal communication). Apart from specialist training for clinical geneticists, postgraduate education is even poorer and constitutes a major barrier to the uptake of genetic services. To improve the teaching of genetics to medical students the college has established a medical genetic education task force, while the confidential enquiry into the quality of counselling should improve postgraduate medical understanding of genetic disorders.

Strategies for reaching targets

Several general strategies are required. National feasibility studies for screening programmes for the presymptomatic diagnosis of late

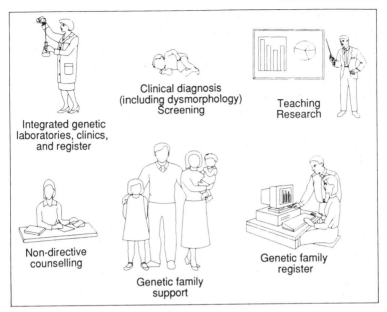

Integrated genetic
laboratories, clinics,
and register

Clinical diagnosis
(including dysmorphology)
Screening

Teaching
Research

Non-directive
counselling

Genetic family
support

Genetic family
register

Functions of the regional genetic services

onset cancers and other genetic diseases should be a high priority. It is hoped that the new central research and development committee[12] will promote genetic programmes of this type. There is also a need to ensure that all appropriate patients have equal access to screening for Down's syndrome and to other well evaluated screening programmes, including those for thalassaemia and Tay-Sachs disease. Additional screening should be introduced for carriers of cystic fibrosis and the fragile X syndrome as soon as these tests have been evaluated. In parallel with these screening programmes there must be study of the social, community, educational, ethical, and logistic issues that may be expected. It will also be important to ensure by medical audit that the highest standards of clinical and laboratory services are achieved and maintained.

The Health of the Nation identifies the "role of the centre to develop new key areas." This is particularly important in medical genetics, which is a new and vulnerable specialty. Regional genetic services must be preserved (figure). This need is recognised by the Royal College of Physicians of London[13] and by other royal colleges and has been endorsed by the Department of Health. It will be extremely damaging to the welfare of patients with genetic disorders and their

175

families, who often live in different health districts, if regional genetic services are splintered by hasty devolution to districts.

In addition to central initiatives, regional genetic committees with multispecialty representation should be charged with strategic planning. They should also provide impartial professional advice to the regional health authority, recommend priorities for developments, and advise on monitoring regionally purchased genetic contracts so as to achieve and maintain an efficient quality service with equal access for patients in all districts.

Advances in medical genetics have implications for other medical specialties. All clinicians should pay increasing attention to this aspect of patient care.

1 Secretary of State for Health. *The health of the nation*. London: HMSO, 1991. (Cm 1523.)
2 Royal College of Physicians of London. *Purchasers' guidelines to genetic services in the NHS. An aid to assessing the genetic services required by the resident population of an average health district*. London: Royal College of Physicians, 1991.
3 Royal College of Physicians of London. *Prenatal diagnosis and genetic screening. Community and service implications*. London: Royal College of Physicians, 1989.
4 Wald N, Cuckle H. Some practical issues in the antenatal detection of neural tube defect and Down's syndrome. In: Owen Drife J, Donnai D, eds. *Antenatal diagnosis of fetal abnormalities*. London: Springer-Verlag, 1991:45-57.
5 Bulow S. Familial polyposis coli. *Dan Med Bull* 1987;**34**:1-15.
6 McKusick VA. The defect in Marfan syndrome. *Nature* 1991;**352**:279-81.
7 Yu S, Pritchard E, Kremer E, Lynch M, Nancarrow J, Baker E, *et al*. Fragile X genotype characterized by an unstable region of DNA. *Science* 1991;**252**: 1179-81.
8 Oberle F, Rousseau D, Heitz D, Kretz C, Devys D, Hanauer A, *et al*. Instability of a 550-base pair DNA segment and abnormal methylation in fragile X syndrome. *Science* 1991;**252**: 1097-102.
9 Rona RJ, Swan AV, Beech R, Prentice L, Wilson OM, Mole G, *et al*. Demand for DNA probe testing in three genetic centres in Britain. (August 1986 to July 1987) *J Med Genet* 1989;**26**:226-36.
10 Conclusions and recommendations. In: Owen Drife J, Donnai D, eds. *Antenatal diagnosis of fetal abnormalities*. London: Springer-Verlag, 1991: 353-5.
11 Royal College of Physicians of London. *Teaching genetics to medical students*. London: Royal College of Physicians, 1990.
12 Peckham M. Research and development for the National Health Service. *Lancet* 1991;**338**: 367-71.
13 Royal College of Physicians of London. *Clinical genetics in 1990 and beyond*. London: Royal College of Physicians, 1991.

Smoking

JACKY CHAMBERS, AMANDA KILLORAN,
ANN McNEILL, DONALD REID

Any government that is seriously committed to improving the health of its population must have a strategy for controlling the use of tobacco and reducing the number of people who smoke. It is therefore encouraging that *The Health of the Nation* recognises smoking as a key area for action and suggests a fairly ambitious target that by the year 2000 around four out of five people should be non-smokers (box).[1]

Our discussion focuses on the relation between smoking and the prevention of disease and, drawing on experience from other countries, whether the measures outlined in the consultation document are likely to be adequate to achieve the smoking target.

Smoking as a key area

The Health of the Nation describes smoking as "the largest single preventable cause of mortality" and adds that "it accounts for more than a third of all deaths in middle age."[1] Current estimates suggest that about 115 000 deaths,[2] and roughly 106 000 admissions to hospital[3] in Britain every year are attributable to smoking. Passive smoking increases the risk of lung cancer by 10-30% and causes respiratory complaints in children.[4]

Smoking costs the NHS at least £500 million annually,[5] but the costs of ill health to society are considerably more, with an estimated 50 million working days being lost through sickness absence.[6] The benefits of giving up smoking in reducing the risks of lung cancer and coronary heart disease for the adult population, including elderly people, are well documented,[7-9] as is the effectiveness of different kinds of interventions at an individual and population level.[10-12]

Another reason for choosing smoking as a key area is the public's strong views on smoking. As Mr Waldegrave points out those steering the future direction of a national health strategy for England "need to take heed of the views of the people who will have to implement it, including the people themselves." Surveys of public opinion suggest that most are in favour of stronger measures to control the advertising of tobacco and restrict smoking in public places. (Office of Population Censuses and Surveys, unpublished data). Furthermore, most (54%) regular adult smokers would like to stop smoking for good (Department of Health, unpublished data) and most young people (88%) believe that breathing other people's smoke is dangerous.[13]

As smoking affects both the quality and the duration of life it could provide a common goal that would bridge the NHS and other agencies. Everyone who works in the NHS, in whatever discipline, comes face to face daily with the harm caused by tobacco smoking; many feel helpless in preventing it. Widespread commitment to a national goal to reduce smoking, especially if this included a clear commitment from the government, could mobilise NHS workers' enthusiasm to work with and alongside other organisations.

Case against smoking as a key area

Efforts to reduce smoking are almost always met with fierce opposition and powerful counter lobbying,[14] most of which originates from the tobacco industry. Attempts to encourage people not to smoke lead to accusations of interference with personal liberties, "nannying," or "victim blaming." Loss of £6 billion revenue from tobacco taxation,[15] increased unemployment, and rising costs to the NHS because of increasing numbers of people surviving beyond the age of 65 years are all arguments which are put forward.

A stronger case is the evidence that smoking provides an essential coping strategy for people whose lives might otherwise be intolerable because of the material and cultural deprivation they experience.[16] Strategies to reduce smoking among these groups would need to tackle the origins and effects of poverty, so why not address these issues first?

Finally, recent falls in the prevalence of smoking might be interpreted as showing that little more needs to be done in the future and greater attention needs to be paid to other areas.

Suggested targets in green paper

To reduce the proportion of men smoking cigarettes to 22% by 2000 and of women to 21% (reductions of 33% and 30% respectively). The target can further be broken down by sex and age group

Age (years)	Men		Women	
	1988 (%)	2000 (%)	1988 (%)	2000 (%)
16-19	28	20	28	20
20-24	37	25	37	25
25-49	37	25	35	25
50-59	33	20	34	20
≥60	26	15	21	15

What should the targets be?

Smoking is the only area where the government is considering targets differentiated by age and sex (but not social class). More than seven million (63%) smokers belong to the manual occupational groups and there are also important geographical variations in smoking prevalence between the north and south of England.[17] These differences in smoking behaviour at least partly explain the gradients in mortality from coronary heart disease observed in different parts of the country.[18] Targets for smoking should be set in ways which will guide national and local prevention strategies. Thus differentiated targets for smoking must take account of the current distribution of smokers in the population and be based on social class or geography.[19]

Between 1982 and 1988 rates of fall in smoking prevalence were around 0·8% a year for men and 0·5% a year for women (about 159 000 fewer smokers a year).[17] The government's target requires a rate of fall of 0·9% a year for men and 0·7% a year for women (or 300 000 fewer smokers) each year. Greater efforts and commitment will undoubtedly be required.

But targets to reduce smoking should not be set in isolation from the rest of the national health strategy. Targets for coronary heart disease, stroke and cancers, as well as for the health of pregnant

179

women are dependent on those for smoking. Much could be learnt from work undertaken in Holland,[20] in which the impact of risk factor reduction on disease mortality has been predicted through statistical modelling techniques.

Towards a future strategy

The Health of the Nation describes two separate strategies for achieving the target: to reduce the number of young people who start to smoke and to encourage current smokers to give up. The measures outlined for achieving this include health promotion by the primary health care team, the adoption of smoking policies governing the workplace and public places; national programmes of health education targeted particularly at teenagers and pregnant women; and controls on tobacco advertising and levels of duty.

International experience

Experience in other countries shows the importance of adopting a comprehensive strategy for tobacco control. In 1988 Californian voters passed the bill "Proposition 99," which introduced a range of measures including an increase in cigarette taxation from $0·10 to $0·35 a pack, the additional revenue being used to fund a $30 million media campaign, tobacco education in schools, and training for physicians. Local bylaws were also passed to protect non-smokers in the workplace. California's Department of Health Services has set a target of reducing the prevalence of smoking by 75% between 1990 and 1999. Since the bill was passed smoking prevalence has dropped from 26·3% (1987) to 21·2% (1990).[21]

Canada also has a national strategy to reduce tobacco use and the federal government has adopted a range of legislative measures to support its implementation. The Tobacco Products Control Act aims at phasing out all tobacco advertising through bill boards, the media, and retail premises by 1993; requires manufacturers to display prominent health warnings on packets; and controls the promotion of brand names through sponsorship agreements.

In 1990 a separate (private members) act, the Non-Smokers Health Act, also came into force. This act requires all employers who run businesses within federal jurisdiction such as banking, broadcasting, and other public services to restrict smoking to separately ventilated rooms or ban it altogether. Smoking is not permitted on intercity buses and will be phased out from all domestic and international

Towards smoking targets for the year 2000

Current	Future
Fiscal policy Ad hoc increases in price of tobacco	Regular increases in the real price of tobacco as a declared policy. Tobacco not included in retail price index
Control in tobacco promotion Broadcasting ban but widespread televising of tobacco sponsored sport Voluntary agreement on control of tobacco advertising but ineffective Strong health warning in line with European Community directive Sales to children under 16 prohibited through legislation – weak enforcement	Complete ban on all forms of tobacco advertising, promotion, and sponsorship, including that for other products bearing the names, logos, and designs of cigarettes, tobacco, or cigar brands Increased size of health warnings. Generic packaging Strict enforcement of under age illegal sales by local authorities including license withdrawal
Smoke free environments Discretionary enforcement of restrictions in public places	Smoking restriction in public places governed by legislation—including schools, health premises, public transport, local authority premises
Health promotion Piecemeal funding of health promotion campaigns Developing local health strategies. Variable collaboration with district and family health services authorities Health promotion in general practitioner contract Health education low priority in school national curriculum	Fully resourced national health promotion programme Smoking designated as joint priority in local health strategies Local targets for recording of smoking status agreed with general practitioners Implementation of personal and social education programmes in national curriculum

flights by 1993. Tobacco taxation has increased since 1984, the sharpest increase being last year when total tax on cigarettes rose from $2·64 to $3·72. Between 1984 and 1989 tobacco consumption per person fell by 29% compared with 5% during the same period in Britain.[22]

Strategy for England

Strategies for health cannot be lifted off the shelf, nor can they be imported. They need to be woven from the cultural, political, and economic fabric of the society for which they are intended.

The pace at which progress can be achieved has to be judged. Public demand for public health measures and the measures' acceptability should be important criteria in determining the pace of change.

181

Research should be done to assess these factors to prevent serious misjudgments occurring when formulating government policy. The health costs of moving too slowly in reducing the prevalence of smoking need to be assessed. In our view the pace of change is currently too slow (box).

The Health of the Nation lists most of the basic ingredients used by other countries to reduce smoking in the population, although it is uncertain which ingredients the government intends to adopt and whether these will go far enough.

Price

Price has a considerable influence on tobacco consumption. For every 1% increase in price controlling for disposable income and other factors, consumption can be expected to fall by 0·5%,[23] this fall being seen particularly among those on low income.[24] *The Health of the Nation* highlights the 15% increase in duty levelled on tobacco products in the 1991 budget and quotes the Chancellor of the Exchequer as saying "there are strong arguments for a big duty increase on tobacco." We estimate that if this rise was reflected in a price increase tobacco consumption would be expected to fall by around 7% more than if the tax duty had remained unchanged.

A recent study for the Health Education Authority analyses the relation between increases in cigarette prices and taxation, other health promotion activities, and consumption, based on the British experience.[25] The results predict that considerable price increases would be required to achieve the government's smoking targets, if this was the only additional measure taken. The same targets could, however, be achieved with much more modest price increases if there was adequate investment in health promotion and strong action on controlling tobacco promotion.

Price increase remains, however, the cornerstone of a future strategy. Indeed if there was a clear commitment to a policy of large, annual increases (in real terms) in tobacco duty for the next 10 years, this could by itself lead to an immediate and sharp drop in smoking prevalence.

Tobacco promotion

Every year the tobacco industry spends around £113m on advertising and promoting their products.[27] The British government has in the past opposed a complete ban on advertising and prefers instead to continue the present system of voluntary controls, or self regulation by the industry. A European Community directive containing new proposals to restrict advertising sponsorship will be debated in November. Meanwhile new voluntary agreements for the United Kingdom have recently been announced; these restrict advertisements and bill boards near schools and playgrounds, tighten up restrictions on cigarette advertisements in women's magazines, reduce the number (but do not specify size) of shopfront advertisements; and require new health warnings but maintain the attribution. The Committee for Monitoring Agreements on Tobacco Advertising and Sponsorship (COMATAS), which comprises equal numbers of representatives from the government and the tobacco industry, monitors whether the agreements are being honoured by the industry.

The basic flaw with a voluntary agreement system is that it leads to a piecemeal approach which is industry led. When steps are taken to tighten up in one way, other ways of promoting tobacco are found. For example, although cigarette advertisements were removed from television in 1965, 65% of children aged between 9 and 15 currently claim to have seen cigarette advertising on television.[27] Women's magazines with a large readership of young women (15-24 years) are not allowed to carry cigarette advertisements. Yet one study estimated that about seven million women in this age group are exposed in this way.[28]

The reasons why children and young people take up smoking are complex[29] and a relation has been shown between awareness of advertising and under age smoking.[30] Peer pressure, parental and sibling smoking, desire to look grown up, and availability are all factors. By the age of 10, more than 28% of children have tried their first cigarette.[13]

Glamorous images of smoking portrayed by the industry undermine the influence of health education in schools and help to create the view that smoking is adult and socially acceptable. If the government is serious about achieving the smoking target and protecting children from the promotion of cigarettes it should support the European Community directive for a ban on advertising in November.

On labelling an important step has already been taken. The new regulations requiring tobacco products to carry hard hitting messages such as smoking kills will come into effect in January 1992 and the attribution of this warning to chief medical officers will be dropped.

The Children and Young Persons (Protection from Tobacco) Act, which increases fines for illegal sales of cigarettes to children and outlaws the sale of single cigarettes, has just been ratified. Its success will depend on proper enforcement of the law at local level. Measures to strengthen its enforcement should be included in a future strategy.

Smoke free environments

At the European Community Council of Health Ministers in May 1989 a mixed resolution was adopted to ban smoking in enclosed public places by legislative or other means, allowing designated zones to be reserved for smokers. Member states are expected to report on progress every two years. The government has so far not favoured legislation as the best way to make progress in Britain. Smoking policies have been introduced into workplaces over the past 10 years. In a survey of the top 500 companies 79% of personnel directors said they had no smoking areas, and 22% said they had complete smoking bans.[31]

In the NHS 166 out of 190 district health authorities had policies governing smoking on NHS premises,[32] whereas less than 10% of primary schools had any policies regulating smoking by staff or by governors (Health Education Authority, unpublished data). Surveys also show that most people, including smokers, favour restricting smoking in places such as restaurants, banks, and post offices and about 60% favour legislation to ban smoking on public transport.[33]

Although some progress is clearly being made, a commitment to legislate for smoke free environments or to strengthen existing legislation could speed up the rate of change. This could be particularly important for workplaces with high proportions of manual, part time, and shift workers, where a majority vote may go against the rights of non-smokers to breathe smoke free air. In particular, there should be a central commitment by all government departments to introduce restrictions on smoking in those public places which fall within their remit.

Health promotion

Public education about smoking is a vital element in achieving the smoking target. The methods available include media campaigns such as advertising on television, radio and television programmes, newspaper and magazine articles and personal or group education by health professionals, teachers, or lay people. National and local media provide cost effective ways of raising awareness and motivating large numbers of people to give up smoking. Several studies suggest that with sufficient investment in media campaigns the prevalence of smoking does fall,[34] although the picture is less positive for teenagers.[35]

In the United Kingdom No Smoking Day achieves 90% awareness among smokers and over 85% among the general population and helps to prompt an estimated 50 000 smokers to give up each year (National No Smoking Day Committee, unpublished data). However, we estimate that at least £10 million a year would need to be invested to provide campaigns that are similar to those found to be effective in other countries. This work would need to be supported by a further £10 million for community based interventions.

Media campaigns can also enhance the impact of direct personal education undertaken locally and bring down smoking rates even further.[34] Analysis of 40 studies confirmed the importance of advice from general practitioners.[9] Frequent, consistent advice given opportunistically can result in around 5% of smokers giving up for more than a year.[36 37] The new general practitioners' contract and the additional investment in health promotion provide a real opportunity to help achieve the smoking target.

However, resources and staff for health promotion during health care need to be deployed flexibly to meet different social needs. Hospital based staff, pharmacists, and many other professionals also have an important part to play. Such people represent trusted and credible sources of information and advice and also come into contact with large numbers of the general public.

At a more strategic level, the new purchasing authorities which were created as a result of the NHS reforms could incorporate into their service specifications and contracts with providers a requirement to provide smoke free environments and patient education on smoking.[38 39] Neighbourhood targets for reducing smoking or intermediate goals towards this aim could be negotiated with service providers, including general practice based teams through purchasing plans developed jointly between family health services authorities, district health authorities, and general practitioner fundholders.

Monitoring and surveillance

Smoking targets are measurable over time both nationally and locally. The general household survey provides data on smoking every two years, and many regions and districts conduct health and lifestyle surveys, which include information about smoking behaviour.[40] Some regions are now in a position to agree local smoking targets with their health authorities. Unfortunately, some of the sampling methods and questions that have been used for these surveys are not standardised so it is difficult to make comparisons over time and between different parts of the country.

Introducing annual reports and computerised data collection systems into general practice and district health authorities makes monitoring local trends in smoking prevalence possible. Central guidance and support on how to collect reliable smoking data at local or practice level would prove useful.

Problems in implementing a smoking strategy

International experience shows that there are no valid reasons why a drop in smoking prevalence to 21% by the year 2000 should not be possible, providing the right measures are taken.

The habit of smoking is undoubtedly associated with the problems of poverty, unemployment, and other kinds of deprivation but there is a worrying tendency for public health activists to use this association as an excuse for inaction. We need to remember that there are still more than 12 million regular cigarette smokers in England (14 million in the United Kingdom), most of whom (61%) are light smokers (<20 cigarettes a day)[17] and do not live in conditions of poverty. Thus the scope for further change is considerable, and most smokers do want to give up.

People who, because of their material or social circumstances, will find it more difficult to give up or indeed stop their children from smoking will need additional help. It is difficult, but possible, to use community based approaches to tackle both the short term problems of smoking and the longer term problems of poverty for those who are most vulnerable to their smoking habit. Another problem is of professionals' lack of confidence that they can make an important contribution. Professional training bodies, colleges, and institutes could do more to help clinicians, nurses, and other staff promote health more effectively.

Surprisingly, NHS managers seem to be unaware that investment in smoking prevention programmes can contribute to their agenda of "health gain," and that patient education on smoking should be provided by all NHS services and not just the staff who work in their health education units.

A different problem is the tendency at national level to think separately about smoking education strategies for children and for adults. Stopping adults from smoking and preventing children from smoking are two sides of the same coin. One cannot be achieved without the other. Investment in health education programmes which are targeted at particular groups will be really cost effective only if they are conducted within the context of a whole population's approach. (Reid D, Killoran A, McNeill A, unpublished work.)

We also need to remember that many of the measures adopted in other countries have come about only as a result of a carefully orchestrated, broadly based health lobby and that the skills to do this in Britain are relatively poorly developed. The institutions and traditions of our professions do not encourage the view that lobbying is part of their job—in fact such behaviour is often frowned on as disruptive and difficult. Contacting the local press, speaking on the radio, and meeting members of parliament or councillors are not skills which are actively developed in training. This is a pity as it is often the younger members of the profession who have the energy and enthusiasm to work towards this kind of goal.

Finally, the additional measures which government itself is prepared to adopt to reduce smoking prevalence should be made explicit in a future white paper—for nowhere is the need for a central role more obvious. Time and effort need to be put into securing the commitment of all government departments to achieving the smoking target, and someone needs to take on responsibility for doing this.

Expectations have been raised by the consultation process, many look forward to seeing what is proposed. For some the measures which are set out for tobacco will be a kind of litmus test of government intent—an important sign that its desire to improve the health of the nation is sincere.

We thank Patti White, Joy Townsend, Christine Godfrey, and Antony Morgan for comments and advice.

1 Secretary of State for Health. *The health of the nation.* London: HMSO, 1991. (Cm 1523.)
2 Currie E. Parliamentary written answer. *House of Commons Official Report (Hansard)* 1987 November 16;**122**:col 280. (No 44.)
3 Roberts JL, Graveling PA, eds. *The big kill: smoking epidemic in England and Wales.* London: Health Education Council, 1985.
4 Independent Scientific Committee on Smoking and Health. *Fourth report.* London: HMSO, 1988.
5 Maynard A, Harchman G, Wheelen A. Data note 9. Measuring the social costs of addictive substances. *Br J Addict* 1987;**82**:701-6.
6 Royal College of Physicians. *Health or smoking?* London: Pitman, 1983.
7 Doll R, Peto R. Mortality in relation to smoking 20 years' observations on male British doctors. *BMJ* 1976;ii:1525-30.

8 Cock DG, Pocock SJ, Shaper AG, Kussick SJ. Giving up smoking and the risk of heart attacks. A report from the British regional heart study. *Lancet* 1986;ii:1376-80.

9 Jajich CL, Ostfeld AM, Freeman DH. Smoking and coronary heart disease—mortality in the elderly. *JAMA* 1984;252:2831-4.

10 Kottke TE, Battista RN, DeFriese GH, Brekke ML. Attributes of successful smoking cessation interventions in medical practice. *JAMA* 1988;259: 2882-9.

11 Fiore M, Novotny TE, Pierce JP, Giovino GA, Hatziandreu EJ, Newcombe PA, *et al.* Methods used to quit smoking in the United States. Do cessation programs help? *JAMA* 1990;263: 2760-5.

12 Pierce J, Macaskill P, Hill D. Long term effectiveness of mass media led anti smoking campaigns in Australia. *Am J Public Health* 1990;80:565-9.

13 Health Education Authority. *Young people's health and lifestyles survey carried out by MORI*. London: HEA (in press).

14 Raw M, White P, McNeill A. *Clearing the air: a guide for action on tobacco*. London: British Medical Association, 1990.

15 Ryder R. Parliamentary written answer. *House of Commons Official Report (Hansard)* 1990 February 8:166:col 713. (No 47.)

16 Graham H. Women's smoking and family health. *Soc Sci Med* 1987;25:47-56.

17 Office of Population of Censuses and Surveys. *General household survey, 1988*. London: HMSO, 1990.

18 Shaper AG, Pocock SJ, Wallar M, Cohen NW, Wale CJ, Thomson AG. British Regional Heart Study: cardiovascular risk factors in middle-aged men in 24 towns. *BMJ* 1981;283:179-86.

19 *Setting targets for coronary heart disease—a discussion document*. London: Health Education Authority, 1990.

20 Gunning-Schepers L. The health benefits of prevention: a simulative approach to health policy. Vol 12. No 1-2. Amsterdam: Elsevier Science, 1989.

21 California Department of Health Services. *Tobacco use in California 1990. A preliminary report documenting the decline of tobacco use*. San Diego: University of San Diego, 1991.

22 Department of National Health and Welfare. *Canadians and smoking: an update*. Canada: Minister of Supply and Services, 1991.

23 Godfrey C, Maynard A. Economic aspects of tobacco use and taxation policy. *BMJ* 1988;297:339-43.

24 Townsend J. Cigarette tax economic welfare and social class patterns of smoking. *Applied Economics* 1987;19:335-65.

25 Townsend J. Economic measures to reduce cigarette smoking in the UK and projections of reduced premature mortality. London: Health Education Authority, 1991.

26 Mgadzah R. Battle lines drawn for smoking war. *Marketing Week* 1988 October 21:23.

27 Roberts JL. *Beating the ban*. London: Health Education Authority, 1990.

28 Amos A. Selling tobacco to children. *BMJ* 1990;301:1173-4.

29 Goddard E. *Why children start smoking*. London: HMSO, 1990.

30 Aitken P. *Pushing smoke*. Copenhagen: World Health Organisation Regional Office for Europe, 1988.

31 *Survey of Britain's personnel directors. Research study conducted for BUPA*. London: MORI, 1990.

32 Batten L. *Managing change—smoking policies in the NHS*. London: Health Education Authority, 1990.

33 Consumers' Association. Passive smoking in public. *Which? Way to Health*. 1991;February:14.

34 Flay BR. Mass media and smoking cessation: a critical review. *Am J Public Health* 1987;77:153-60.

35 Bauman KE, LaPrelle J, Brown JD, Koch GG, Padge HCA. The influence of three mass media campaigns on variables related to adolescent cigarette smoking: results of a field experiment. *Am J Public Health* 1991;81:597-604.

36 Russell MAH, Wilson C, Taylor C, Baker CD. Effect of GPs advice against smoking. *BMJ* 1979;ii:231-5.

37 Jamrozcik RK, Veney M, Fowler G, Wald N, Parker G, Van Vunakis H. Controlled trial of three different anti-smoking interventions in general practice. *BMJ* 1984;288:1499-503.

38 Health Education Authority. *NHS white paper. Implications for health promotion/disease prevention*. London: HEA, 1990.

39 Killoran AJ. A healthy start? *Health Services Journal* 1991;29 August:14-6.

40 Health Education Authority/Office of Population Censuses and Surveys. *Health and lifestyle surveys*. London: HEA, 1990.

Poverty

TONY DELAMOTHE

Although *The Health of the Nation* never considers making social inequalities in health a key area, it acknowledges the effects of "social circumstances" and the "physical and social environment" on health and accepts that health varies "significantly" according to social and occupational group.[1] It even provides two examples. Given the usual official reticence on the topic this represents progress.

In his foreword Mr Waldegrave goes a step further: he accepts that remedial measures work. Providing financial support for certain groups and putting a decent home within the reach of every family is partly justified by "their relation to health." But the document backs down from the obvious next step: tackling social inequalities in health head on. Instead it counsels "tempering idealism with pragmatism" when confronting the challenge of the variations. "The Government does not believe there is any panacea—here or elsewhere in the world—either in terms of a full explanation or a single action which will eradicate the problem." Progress may be possible on three fronts:

- Through the continued general pursuit of greater economic prosperity and social wellbeing
- Through trying to increase understanding of the variations and the action which might effectively address them
- Through specific initiatives to address the health needs of particular groups.

In his valedictory report on the state of the public health the last chief medical officer wrote that low income, unhealthy behaviour, and poor housing and environmental amenities had the clearest links with the excess burden of ill health.[2] At the press conference launching his

189

report Sir Donald was more forthright, saying that health inequalities will be eradicated only by government measures to tackle poverty and improve the conditions in which people live. "While to specialists in public health the most attractive points of initial attack are health promotion initiatives to reduce risk factors such as smoking, poor diet, and physical activity, there is a limit to the extent to which such improvements are likely to occur in the absence of a wider strategy to change the circumstances in which these risks arise by reducing deprivation and improving physical environment."[3]

Social inequalities in health must therefore warrant further scrutiny as a possible key area.

Major cause of ill health

The Health of the Nation recommends judging candidates for key area status against three criteria. How do social inequalities in health measure up? The first criterion is that the area should be a major cause of premature death or avoidable ill health in the population as a whole or among specific groups. Examining "burdens of disease"—mortality, morbidity, and cost —is one way suggested for identifying the most serious problems.

Mortality

A gap exists between the death rates of non-manual and manual workers for most causes of death in almost every age group, and the gap is widening (figs 1 and 2[4]). In 1981, 62 of the 66 "major list" causes of death in men were more common in social classes IV and V (combined) than in other classes. Of the 70 major causes of death in women, 64 were more common in women married to men in social classes IV and V.[5]

Stillbirths, deaths within the first year of life, and deaths in children are all more common in the lower socioeconomic groups (fig 1). If the whole population had experienced the same death rates as the non-manual classes there would have been 700 fewer stillbirths and 1500 fewer deaths in the first year of life in England and Wales in 1988,[6] 750 fewer deaths in children in England and Wales in 1981,[7] and 17 000 fewer deaths in men aged 20-64 in Great Britain in 1981.[8]

The Health of the Nation also suggests using less "crude" measures of mortality, such as "years of life lost." When this is done the familiar socioeconomic gradient reappears, although it is steeper than for the

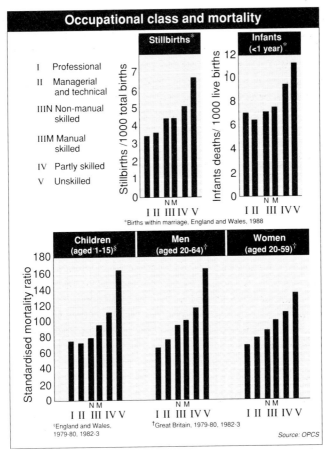

Figure 1—Occupational class and mortality in babies and adults

standardised mortality ratio (table I). It has also increased between 1971 and 1981.[9]

Morbidity

Data from the general household surveys show a difference in the prevalence of longstanding illness between manual and non-manual groups, which has increased between 1980 and 1988.[10] Clear socio-economic gradients exist for the commonest reported causes of longstanding illness: musculoskeletal, circulatory, and respiratory conditions.[2] Davey Smith and colleagues cite numerous studies that

191

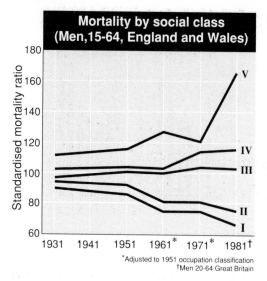

Figure 2—Mortality by social class in men aged 15-64, England and Wales

have been published since the Black report that show social class differentials in morbidity.[11] Less privileged groups therefore not only have a shorter life span but also spend more of their lives in poor health.

Effective interventions

The second criterion is that effective interventions to improve health should be possible. The gap between the pay of the highest and lowest paid is now greater than at any time since official records began

TABLE I—Comparison of social class differences in years of potential life lost (per 1000 population) and standardised mortality ratio; 1981 data for Great Britain[9]

	Men aged 20-64		Women aged 20-59	
	Years of potential life lost	Standardised mortality ratio	Years of potential life lost	Standardised mortality ratio
Social class:				
I	39	66	16	69
II	45	76	18	78
III Non-manual	57	94	22	87
III Manual	63	106	23	100
IV	72	116	27	110
V	114	165	34	134
Ratio of classes V:I	2·9	2·5	2·1	1·9

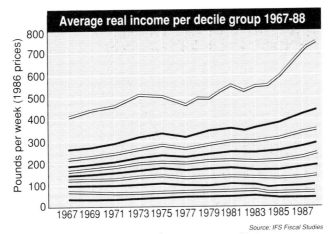

Figure 3—Average real income per decile group, 1967-88

in 1886 (fig 3).[12] [13] The widening gap continues a trend that began during the 1979-81 recession after several decades of stable pay differentials.

With the widening gap in pay came a massive increase in the number of relatively poor people. The number of people living on less than half the average income—the European Community's definition of poverty[14]—more than doubled between 1979 and 1988, regardless of whether disposable income was assessed before or after the deduction of housing costs (table II).[15] Depending on the definition used either one in four or one in five children was living below the poverty line in 1988.

Although real income grew by about one third for the whole population between 1979 and 1988, the median income (after deduction of housing costs) of people in the lowest two deciles of

TABLE II—Number (percentage) of people living on less than half average income (Great Britain)[15]

	All	Children
	Before deduction of housing costs	
1979	3 750 000 (7·1)	1 310 000 (9·8)
1988	9 130 000 (16·8)	2 530 000 (21·1)
	After deduction of housing costs	
1979	4 930 000 (9·4)	1 620 000 (12·2)
1988	11 750 000 (21·6)	3 010 000 (25·1)

the income distribution increased by only 2% and 5%—hardly the "trickledown" that was predicted. In the United States, whose economic policies Britain's most resembled in the 1980s, the same thing happened: "the rich got richer and the poor got poorer," the numbers in poverty increased, and trickledown similarly failed to materialise.[16] This must cast some doubt on the assertion that "the continued general pursuit of greater economic prosperity and social well being" necessarily leaves everyone better off.

One of the government's responses to social inequalities has been to target financial help to those in greatest need, and the benefit system was revised in 1988 to facilitate this. Whether the change is achieved this goal will have to await analysis of the next *Households Below Average Income*, which is unlikely to be published before next year. Early figures suggest that uptake of the new benefits has been no better than for those they replaced. Even for families receiving their full entitlement the adequacy of the new benefits has been repeatedly questioned. Agencies such as Barnado's, Child Poverty Action Group, National Associations of Citizen's Advice Bureaux, and National Children's Home doubt that the 1988 changes did anything to improve the conditions of those most in need.

Clearly the current arrangements are failing children, who can hardly be blamed for the circumstances in which they find themselves. Common decency justifies attempts to improve their welfare now. But evidence has also been accumulating that socioeconomic circumstances in childhood may affect the development of diseases in later life,[17 18] doubly justifying efforts to improve children's lot.

With substantially more benefits unlikely to be available for the needy, what interventions offering "significant scope for improvement in health" are possible? Quick and Wilkinson suggest a way forward.[19 20] On the basis of recent research they argue that overall health standards in developed countries are more dependent on the distribution of income within a population than with its average level. The most effective way of improving health is therefore to make incomes more equal. In the nine developed countries for which data are comparable life expectancy is closely correlated with the distribution of income (defined as the proportion of total income after tax and benefit income received by the least well off 70%). Their findings suggest that two thirds of the variation in life expectancy between these countries is related to differences in income distribution.

Redistributing income to offset the health disadvantage experienced by the poor would therefore be the best way of improving the average standard of health. Because in developed countries increases in income produce sharply diminishing health returns redistributing income from the relatively rich to the relatively poor might have little negative effect on the health of the better off.

Supporting evidence comes from a comparison between Britain and Japan. At the beginning of the 1970s income distribution and life expectancy were quite similar. Japan now has the most equally distributed income in the world—and the longest life expectancy.[21] Further evidence comes from Britain during both world wars. Paradoxically, civilian life expectancy increased two to three times faster in wartime than during the rest of the century. Both wars were periods of rapid income redistribution. More recently—as Britain has become a much less equal society—mortality in men aged 15-44 has begun increasing (even after excluding deaths from AIDS).[2]

Setting targets and monitoring progress

The third government criterion is that it should be possible to set objectives and to monitor progress towards their achievement. If the objective is to reduce social inequalities in health, what should the targets be? One could be to reduce the social class gradients in mortality and morbidity (measured as the ratio of morbidity or mortality experienced by different classes—either V:I or manual:non-manual).

Analyses of deaths by occupational group are available only every 10 years—too long to wait to check progress. Socioeconomic data on stillbirths and deaths in infants under 1 year are available annually (although with a two and a half year delay) and could be used. Among the various measures available postneonatal mortality (deaths between 28 days and one year) is regarded as the most sensitive to socioeconomic factors. What may muddy the waters is the NHS Management Executive's decision to make variations in infant mortality one of its two main targets this year. Infant mortality would become less useful as a proxy for the health of the whole population if extra resources were being devoted to it.

Another proxy measure—perhaps the least amenable to "interference"—might be mortality in men aged 15-44, particularly since it has been increasing recently. Figures for mortality by age and sex are available with the least delay of all the potentially useful demographic variables.

Morbidity may respond more rapidly than mortality to interventions, although morbidity lacks the unambiguity of death. For example, differences in "illness behaviour" among socioeconomic groups might invalidate the use of responses to the general household survey, visits to doctors, or absenteeism from work as reliable indicators of morbidity. More detailed studies that have attempted to validate subjective measures with objective indicators of morbidity have been done, although regular studies of sufficient size would be extremely expensive. Perhaps the government's programme of national health surveys will provide more details on how morbidity varies by socioeconomic group, although resources are apparently posing problems.

The case against

Why not make social inequalities a key area, Mr Waldegrave was asked at the press conference marking the publication of *The Health of the Nation*. Wasn't reducing inequalities in health between and within countries the first and possibly most important target of the World Health Organisation's European strategy for Health for All by the Year 2000? (Britain signed up with the strategy in 1985: *The Health of the Nation* may be seen as the government's belated response to national target setting.)

Mr Waldegrave replied that although reducing inequalities in health was "a perfectly legitimate target," the divisions were so fundamental, complicated, long lasting, and recalcitrant that they were not a suitable government target. Targets needed to be specific, measurable, and most of all achievable—"otherwise the whole thing comes into disrepute."

None of these reasons for rejection stands up to scrutiny. Reducing inequalities may be difficult but not impossible. Britain has already managed it during two world wars; Japan managed it over the past 20 years. Sweden's social class differentials in health may persist after 50 years of effort to reduce them, but they are less than Britain's.[22]

The exact mechanisms linking social inequality and poor health may remain poorly understood, but action doesn't need to await fuller understanding. The accurate identification of the organism responsible for cholera epidemics was not necessary for effective preventive action. Identifying the carcinogens in tobacco smoke wasn't a prerequisite for reducing cigarette smoking.

What should the strategy be?

We need government policies on benefits and taxation that would result in more equally distributed incomes. If this sounds like some Scandinavian (or worse, Stalinist) social engineering it's as well to recall that the sudden widening in the distribution of income (fig 3) and the sudden increase in relative poverty since 1979 (table II) flowed directly from government policies and was not a "natural" phenomenon.

The government's policies on taxation have meant that all income groups pay less direct tax now than they would have done in 1979, although the highest tax payers have benefited disproportionately. Of the £28.7bn tax cuts made between 1978-9 and 1991-2, £480m (1·7%) has gone to the 3·7 million taxpayers earning less than £5000 a year whereas £9500m (33%) has gone to the 400 000 people earning over £50 000 a year.[23]

The main factor in the increased numbers of people living in relative poverty was the government's decision in 1980 to index social security benefits to prices rather than to earnings. Since 1979 the relative value of retirement pensions, unemployment benefit, and invalidity benefit has fallen by one fifth compared with average earnings.[24]

John Hills has calculated that since 1979 the changes in direct taxation and benefits have been achieved at virtually zero net cost. "The cuts in direct taxes have been entirely paid for by the cuts in the generosity of benefits . . . the overwhelming majority of the bottom half . . . have lost; the overwhelming majority of the top 30% have gained."[25]

What of poor housing's "clear link" with the excess burden of ill health?[2 26] The government has discouraged building of new council houses (new starts are down by three quarters since 1979) and encouraged the sale of existing council houses. High interest rates, recession, and unemployment have taken their toll: mortgage repossessions and households accepted as homeless are both at record highs. Government policies have been responsible for this: government policies could just as easily reverse these trends. The government provides some £7bn in mortgage relief, which goes to the relatively better off. (In 1988-9 the estimated cost of the relief was equivalent to nearly three quarters of the total public expenditure on housing, including housing benefit.[27]) Expenditure on mortgage relief could easily be diverted to better housing for the poor.

Problems of implementation

The problem of making social inequalities of health a key area is that the solutions lie beyond the Department of Health, and the omens for interdepartmental cooperation are not good. Mr Waldegrave may be reluctant to tackle social inequalities in health; some of his colleagues seem unaware of any connection between socioeconomic circumstances and health (fig 4). As Wilkinson says, "the Chancellor has a much greater impact on health than the Secretary of State for Health, a thought that may well not cross the minds of either."[19]

The sad fact is that the first aim of political parties is to get elected (or re-elected) to government. Reversing the tax cuts of high earners and abolishing mortgage relief could be political suicide for whichever party proposed it.

Convincing enough people of the benefits of income redistribution will be difficult if not impossible. (Haven't the poor always been with us?) The first step must be to emphasise that there is nothing "natural" about the current state of affairs: it results from political choices. Choices could be different, and changing government policy need not necessarily spell industrial ruin. In fact, it could mean the opposite: look at egalitarian, long living Japan or the work of Alesina and Rodrik, who found that among democracies more equal income distribution was associated with higher growth rates.[28]

If the health of the nation—the whole nation—is to improve then the distribution of the disposable income of its population needs to be made more equal. Establishing a classless society would not neces-

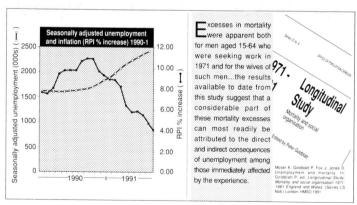

Figure 4—Come on down: the price is right

sarily produce this outcome, although it would vastly increase the
likelihood of doing so.

1 Secretary of State for Health. *The health of the nation*. London: HMSO, 1991. (Cm 1523.)
2 Chief Medical Officer. *On the state of the public health 1990*. London: HMSO, 1991.
3 Brindle D. Medical chief urges anti-poverty fight. *Guardian* 1991 Sept 13:4(cols 1-3).
4 Wilkinson RG. *Class and health: research and longitudinal data*. London: Tavistock, 1986.
5 Jacobson B, Smith A, Whitehead M. *The nation's health: a strategy for the 1990s*. London: King's Fund, 1991.
6 Office of Population Censuses and Surveys. *Mortality statistics: perinatal and infant: social and biological factors 1988*. London: HMSO, 1991. (Series DH3 No 22.)
7 Office of Population Censuses and Surveys. *Occupational mortality: childhood supplement 1979-80, 1982-83*. London: HMSO: 1988. (Series DS No 8.)
8 Office of Population Censuses and Surveys. *Occupational mortality: decennial supplement 1979-80, 1982-83*. London: HMSO, 1986. (Series DS No 2.)
9 Blane D, Davey Smith G, Bartley M. Social class differences in years of potential life lost: size, trends, and principal causes. *BMJ* 1990;**301**:429-32.
10 Chief Medical Officer. *On the state of the public health 1989*. London: HMSO, 1990.
11 Davey Smith G, Bartley M, Blane D. The Black report on socioeconomic inequalities in health 10 years on. *BMJ* 1990;**301**:373-7.
12 Jenkins SP. Income inequality and living standards. *Fiscal Studies* 1991;**12**: 1-28.
13 Huhne C. Pay gap "widest since 1886." *Independent on Sunday* 1991 Sept 29:3(col 6).
14 European Commission. *Final report on the second European poverty programme*. Brussels: European Commission, 1991. (Com(91)29.)
15 Social Security Committee. *Low income statistics: households below average income tables 1988*. London: HMSO, 1991.
16 Prowse M. Buddy, can you still spare a dime. *Financial Times* 1991 5-6 Oct:VIII(col 1-7).
17 Baird D. Environment and reproduction. *Br J Obstet Gynaecol* 1985;**82**:115-21.
18 Barker DJP. The fetal and infant origins of adult disease. *BMJ* 1990;**301**:1111.
19 Quick A, Wilkinson R. *Income and health*. London: Socialist Health Association, 1991.
20 Wilkinson RG. Income distribution and life expectancy. *BMJ* (in press).
21 Marmot MG, Davey Smith G. Why are the Japanese living longer? *BMJ* 1989;**299**:1547-51.
22 Vagero D, Lundberg O. Health inequalities in Britain and Sweden. *Lancet* 1989;ii:35-6.
23 Maude F. Written answers. *House of Commons Official Report (Hansard)* 1991 May 9;190: cols 552-4. (No 104.)
24 Rowthorn B. Government spending and taxation in the Thatcher era. In: Michie J, ed. *The economic legacy: 1979-1992*. London: Academic Press (in press).
25 Hills J. *Changing tax: how the tax system works and how to change it*. London: CPAG, 1990.
26 Lowry S. *Housing and health*. London: *BMJ*, 1991;**303**:838-40.
27 Hills J, Mullings B. Housing: a decent home for all at a price within their means? In: Hills J, ed. *The state of welfare: the welfare state in Britain since 1974*. Oxford: Clarendon Press, 1990.
28 Alesina A, Rodrik D. *Distributive politics and economic growth*. York: Centre for Economic Policy Research, 1991. (Discussion paper No 565.)

Illegal drugs

JOHN STRANG

The war on drugs will never be won, just as the war on cancer and the war on poverty will never be won; but what folly to fail to identify achievable goals, measures of progress, and strategy of action in the ongoing war. In each of these unwinnable wars great benefit (to both personal and public health) may be accrued from fighting on the right fronts. The challenge for the strategist is to direct the available resources so as to make advances on key fronts while guarding against damaging losses elsewhere.

Does injecting drug use really deserve to be included as one of the identified key areas? Considerations of health strategy have previously been distorted by prejudice and political sensitivities—and it is difficult to believe that the new association with HIV and AIDS will improve the clarity of vision. But we must now address the synergistic pathology of drug misuse and HIV,[1][2] and we have a right to expect more from a government which has described drug misuse as "the greatest peace-time threat to our nation"[3] and HIV and AIDS as "the greatest new threat to public health this century."[4] By 1986 official guesstimates were of 75 000-150 000 opiate misusers, half of whom were believed already to be injecting, plus a similar number of amphetamine injectors.[1] Like it or not, injecting drug misuse will have a profound impact on the future health of the nation.

For most diseases, there is a degree of stability in the extent of penetration through society. This is not true for either drug misuse or HIV infection, and the next few years present an opportunity to influence the rate and extent of spread of injecting drug misuse and HIV infection. Future generations will hold us accountable for the extent of our actions and inactions.

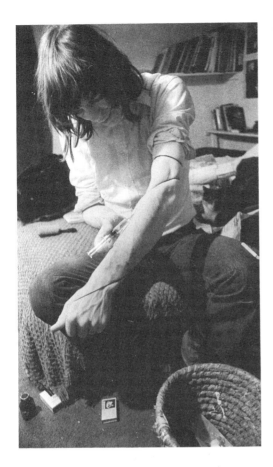

We must put aside morality and focus on harm caused by injecting drugs

Why drug misuse should be a key area

Injecting drug misusers already comprise the fastest growing group of people with AIDS in Europe.[5] Between 1985 and 1989 the proportion of drug injectors among people with newly diagnosed AIDS in Europe rose from 15% to 36%, with the figure rising above 50% in some regions.[6] In England we are fortunate that the epidemic began later than in other countries: hence we have an opportunity to identify targets and work towards improvements which reduce the speed and eventual penetration of HIV and many other future viruses. We missed the opportunity with hepatitis B virus. Are we going to miss it also with HIV?

The shortlist of possible key areas is considered according to three criteria: that the area is a major cause of concern, that there is scope for improvement, and that targets can be set. Drug misuse and HIV are clearly a cause for concern. The scope for improvement is striking when one considers that the most modest of modifications in human behaviour remain our most effective defence against the transmission of HIV (and hepatitis B and C viruses) among and beyond injecting drug users. But it is likely that it is in setting targets that this area is deemed to fail to make the grade, at least for the faint hearted. In fact targets can be set and are essential for a modern well planned strategy—I have outlined them later in this paper.

Are there sufficient opportunities for influencing the condition? Surely the nature of injecting drug use is such that it is a closet behaviour. Perhaps so, but sufficient opportunities already exist, even before its inclusion in a strategy document. General practitioners already see an estimated 6000-9000 opiate addicts every month.[7] Pharmacists are asked for needles and syringes by an estimated 20 000 drug misusers a month.[8] Of the 50 000 inmates in Britain's prisons at any one time, 10% of men and 25% of women will be opiate addicts,[9] although prison medical officers seem to identify such addiction in only 1000 a year.[10]

A distinctive feature of injecting drug use is the extent to which it changes over time. The Home Office figures (2000 addicts in 1970, 6000 in 1980, and 17 000 in 1990)[10] suggest relentless progression, in the face of which any health strategy might be futile. But there is relief, both topographical and emotional. More careful study of the data reveals an epidemic of oral and intravenous amphetamine misuse with substantial psychiatric morbidity in the late 1960s that was effectively countered by public health measures,[11] an intravenous barbiturate epidemic in the 1970s that was associated with high morbidity and mortality,[12 13] and widespread popularity of intravenous Diconal (dipipanone/cyclizine) with its own morbidity that was reversed by new legislation. Even with heroin use the pattern has changed: the universal injection of heroin during the 1960s and 1970s altered during the 1980s, at least in some British cities. By 1987, 90% of heroin users in the Wirrall, Merseyside, were taking heroin by "chasing the dragon,"[14] as were 50% of a local treatment sample in south London;[15] whereas elsewhere (for example, Edinburgh) injecting remained the only route.[16 17] It is this temporal and geographical variation which should inform the targets, the strategy, and the measures of progress.

Case against key area status

There are perhaps two main arguments why injecting drug misuse may not be suitable as a key area. Neither argument is sufficient to make the case. Firstly, there needs to be a clear description of the area, and, with drugs, this is difficult to define. Is it opiate use? Is it illegal behaviour? Is it addiction? These confusions have created mayhem and held back the subject for too long. Sweep aside the moralising and shift the focus to the harm which results (or might result) from use of drugs. Thus the 1981 report from the World Health Organisation considered "hazardous use" (where harm might occur) and "harmful use" (where harm has occurred).[18] In Britain, the 1984 report on prevention identified two legitimate goals: prevention of drug use and prevention of harm associated with drug use.[19] More recently "harm minimisation" has become a new buzz word in the specialty of drugs.[20] Harm minimisation refers to approaches that reduce or remove the harm associated with drug use or with particular aspects of drug taking behaviour. More recently, AIDS has brought a particular clarity to this consideration. The proposed key area is not defined by drug group, nor by legal status of the drug or drug use; it is defined by the nature of harm related to drug use and, in particular, injecting.

The second argument against inclusion is based on the inadequate state of existing means of measurement. Perhaps the government is daunted at the prospect after the dismal response from some district health authorities to the drug "Domesday book" collated by the Department of Health.[21] But this was a bottom up approach designed to chart the territory, whereas *The Health of the Nation* is intended to be a top down strategy.[4] The argument is only as valid as the inability to identify targets and introduce appropriate measures. Targets have already been proposed for HIV and AIDS[22]: targets for injecting drug misuse are proposed below.

Identifying the targets

Despite the neglect of drug misuse in the green paper (box) targets can be set. The opening recommendation from the Department of Health and Social Security's guidelines is that "all doctors have a responsibility to provide care for both the general health needs of drug misusers and their drug related problems."[23] The 1988 Watkins report (part of the United States presidential commission on the HIV epidemic) made important recommendations on targets, such as the

203

Green paper view on drug misuse

The green paper mentions reducing drug misuse only in the context of HIV and AIDS. No specific targets are suggested nor any methods for reducing the prevalence of injecting drug misuse.

---

call for there to be "treatment on demand."[24] The 1988 British report on AIDS and drug misuse made specific recommendations—for example, that "a pattern of community based services should be available in each health district" and that "all GPs should provide care and advice for drug-misusing patients to help them move away from behaviour which may result in them acquiring or spreading the virus."[1] The United States report *Healthy People 2000* went one step further and set the targets that at least 90% of cities should have outreach programmes to deliver HIV risk reduction messages to drug injectors and that at least 75% of primary care providers should "screen for alcohol and other drug problems and provide counselling and referral as needed."[24] I will consider separately general health care targets and drug related targets.

General health targets

Injecting drug use is associated not only with addiction but with other important public health problems such as hepatitis B virus and HIV and AIDS. Currently less than half of some injecting populations are infected with hepatitis B virus. The Department of Health's own report on immunisation recommends that immunisation for injecting drug users should be considered,[26] but remains extremely rare in British drug services.[27] Consider that the Australian strategy document recommends a target of 95% for hepatitis B virus vaccination in at risk groups.[28]

HIV seroprevalence in most British populations of drug injectors is still low (<10%). The chief medical officer's statement about the shifting cost-benefit balance of HIV testing has not been heard yet by drug users or drug workers. Most services are not yet geared up to provide easy access to testing. In house facilities for monitoring of immune status are even rarer. This would not matter if drug users travelled to available HIV services; unfortunately, they do not. Consequently there is a need to set a target similar to that in the

American strategy document: that 80% of all HIV positive people should have been tested.[25]

Treatment capture

But all these targets are set against a shifting baseline, so simple descriptions of volume are inadequate. If drug services are to be given the target of capturing drug addicts at an earlier stage then direct evidence should be sought. Instead of the present practice of presenting data on the age, sex, ethnic distribution, etc (from which changes in capture potential are optimistically deduced) why not go for the real measures? Thus for new patients the interval between addiction and first treatment contact should be measured. Opiate addicts have typically been using drugs on a daily dependent basis for four years before first treatment contact.[29] We should examine measures of this addiction to treatment interval among patients presenting for first treatment, or measures of relapse to treatment interval among returning patients. For the new syringe exchange schemes the drug user has typically been injecting for seven years before first attendance[30]; the equivalent measures would be injecting to exchange interval for new attenders and relapse to exchange interval for reattenders.

Retention

If treatment is believed to be of benefit then the patient must attend long enough for treatment to be administered. Existing measures of retention in programmes are adequate in some areas such as the new syringe exchange schemes[30] but need to be extended to other forms of treatment. More than a third of attenders at most syringe exchange schemes will attend only once, and only one third attend more than five times.[30] Recent small scale studies show a similarly disappointing drop out rate from inpatient[31] and outpatient detoxification programmes.[32] The more widespread and uniform examination of programme retention rates is a simple but essential measure which is surely a prerequisite to competent planning of health care.

Throughput

Laudable and influential as such recommendations may have been, they relate to process not outcome. Indeed the AIDS and drug misuse report draws attention to this point in the section discussing syringe exchange schemes: while such schemes should not be judged wholly on short term results, "ultimately they must be judged on lasting evidence on behaviour change."[1] If the new services are to concern themselves with capture and retention, they must also address throughput (the extent to which the treatment population is changed as a result of the treatment contact)[33].

And so it is to outcome measures that our attention should turn. Abstinence is not the only valid outcome. It is not even the most important (except that it may vary with other outcomes). Key intermediate goals can be identified, such as the move from injecting to oral drug use.[1] (Similar changes away from injecting may also occur outside treatment (for example, from injecting heroin to chasing the dragon),[34] but we are unclear about the part played by health care services). From the point of view of transmission of HIV and other viruses the pure target would be to reduce sharing of injecting equipment. However, measurement would be largely reliant on self reporting, which is unacceptable. So the surrogate target of reduction of injecting should be considered, which is not only more measurable but is also more widely relevant to other harms (for example, overdose). The value of the service would then be gauged according to the extent to which it promoted this reduction—either by stopping non-injectors from starting injecting or by assisting injectors to stop injecting. Simple measures can be used initially. For opiate addicts in a methadone treatment programme, stopping or reducing heroin use has long been used as a measure in the United States; this is measured by the proportion of "dirty" urines detected on random urine testing.[35 36] The proportion of patients with fresh venepuncture marks would be a similar measure. In future a more valuable long term perspective on behaviour change may be obtained from hair analysis.[37]

The strategy almost exists

Perhaps the official strategy document is the government's *Tackling Drug Misuse*, but this document is mainly concerned with customs and excise, police, and other control strategies.[38] The real strategy documents have come from the Advisory Council on the Misuse of Drugs (an independent body set up under the Misuse of Drugs Act 1971). Their reports on treatment and rehabilitation,[39] prevention,[19] and AIDS and drug misuse[12] have received both covert and overt endorsement from the government, and have become the blueprints for subsequent developments of services.

These reports provided a framework for the promotion of involvement by general practitioners, backed up by a local drug service or community drug team in every district.[40 41] Central funding initiatives from the Department of Health pump primed these developments — eventually to the tune of £17m annually.[42] With the AIDS and drug misuse reports, concern shifted from dependent addicts to injecting users — and simultaneously the sought after change in behaviour itself changed. "There is an urgent need for injecting drug users to travel hastily down the section of the road from 'injecting' to 'no injecting.' As a second best, they may make the journey from 'at-risk injecting' to 'safer injecting' insofar as the latter place may exist."[43] From this new perspective, abstinence would perhaps be seen as just a variant on oral only use, but with uncertain robustness and representing an uncertain drain of resources.

In Scotland the early McClelland report identified essential components of a national strategy: "All drug misusers must be brought into contact... [with] a framework of service provisions which offer a comprehensive approach to the many complicated social, financial, legal, psychiatric and other problems which afflict many misusers"; "substitution prescribing is likely to be a necessary part of the means used to attract clients to services and to establish safer drug taking practices"; "practical steps must be taken to provide sterile injecting equipment to addicts who are unwilling to stop injecting"; "staff working with drug misusers will require adequate training and continuing access to sources of expert support...."[44] The "end" becomes the reduction of HIV transmission among drug injectors and, through them, to the broader general public: the "means" becomes the refocusing of any and every possible point of contact with the injector.

Problems with implementation

Unfortunately, these blueprints contain goals but no specific targets or means of measuring progress. Some data on opiate addicts do exist in the Home Office addicts index, and despite continued poor compliance by doctors[45 46] the index has been a valuable indicator of change.[47] The new regional databases[48] (anonymised data on local drug users in contact with statutory and statutorily funded services) should provide the means for implementing many of the necessary measures — for example, measuring changes over time in the addiction to treatment interval of new patients.

Information will still be missing on patterns and extent of drug use outside treatment services. One day (perhaps today) Britain will need to tackle seriously this gap in our information. The United States National Institute on Drug Abuse has for many years conducted household surveys to gather information on different types of drug use "ever" and "last month." *Healthy People 2000* relies heavily on this source of information to gauge the impact of public health and education measures.[25] Until we set up such regular household surveys we will remain in the dark about the worth (or otherwise) of various antidrug of anti-injecting campaigns.

Conclusion

A national health strategy which fails to address specifically the area of injecting drug use is surely a strategy driven by political or public sensitivities, not science. As with HIV and AIDS we will have failed to grasp the nettle if we wait for a time when political and public opinion are calmer or when scientific study is more complete. The extent and nature of the area of injecting drug misuse is changing now: it represents an excellent opportunity to apply a truly valuable strategic approach to the health of the nation.

1 Advisory Council on the Misuse of Drugs. *Report on AIDS and drug misuse.* Part 1. London: HMSO, 1988.
2 Advisory Council on the Misuse of Drugs. *Report on AIDS and drug misuse.* Part 2. London: HMSO, 1989.
3 House of Commons. *Fifth report from the home affairs committee: misuse of hard drugs (interim report).* London: HMSO, 1985.
4 Secretary of State for Health. *The health of the nation.* London: HMSO, 1991. (Cm 1523.)
5 Carballo M, Rezza G. AIDS, drug misuse and the global crisis. In: Strang J, Stimson G, eds. *AIDS and drug misuse: the challenge for policy and practice in the 1990s.* London: Routledge, 1990:16-26.
6 World Health Organisation. AIDS Surveillance in Europe. Geneva: World Health Organisation, 1990. (Quarterly report No 20.)
7 Glanz A, Taylor C. Findings of a national survey of the role of general practitioners in the treatment of opiate misuse: extent of contact with opiate misusers. *BMJ* 1986;**293**:427-30.
8 Glanz A, Bryne C, Jackson P. Role of community pharmacies in prevention of AIDS among injecting drug misusers: findings of a survey in England and Wales. *BMJ* 1989;**299**:1076-9.
9 Maden A, Swinton M, Gunn J. Drug dependence in prisoners *BMJ* 1991;**302**:880.
10 Home Office. *Statistics on the misuse of drugs, 1990.* London: HMSO, 1991.
11 De Alarcon R. An epidemiological evaluation of a public health measure aimed at reducing the availability of methylamphetamine. *Psychol Med* 1972;**2**: 293-300.
12 Ghodse AH. Casualty departments and the monitoring of drug dependence. *BMJ* 1977;i: 1381-2.
13 Jameson A, Glanz A, MacGregor S. *Dealing with drug misuse: crisis intervention in the city.* London: Tavistock, 1984.
14 Parker H, Newcombe R, Bakx KM. The new heroin users: prevalence and characteristics in Wirrall, Merseyside. *Br J Addict* 1987;**82**:147-58.
15 Gossop M, Griffiths P, Strang J. Chasing the dragon: characteristics of heroin chasers. *Br J Addict* 1988;**83**:1159-62.

16 Brettle RP, Bisset K, Burns S, Davidson J, Davidson SJ, Gray JMN, *et al.* Human immunodeficiency virus and drug misuse—the Edinburgh experience. *BMJ* 1987;**295**:421-4.

17 Robertson R. The Edinburgh epidemic: a case study. In: Strang J, Stimson G, eds. *AIDS and drug misuse: the challenge of policy and practice in the 1990s.* London: Routledge, 1990.

18 Edwards G, Arif A, Hodgson R. Nomenclature and classification of drug and alcohol-related problems: a WHO memorandum. *Bull World Health Organ* 1981;**59**:225-42.

19 Advisory Council on the Misuse of Drugs. *Report on prevention.* London: HMSO, 1984.

20 Buning E. The role of harm-reduction programmes in curbing the spread of HIV by drug injectors. In: Strang J, Stimson G, eds. *AIDS and drug misuse: the challenge for policy and practice in the 1990s.* London: Routledge, 1990:153-61.

21 Department of Health and Social Security. *Drug misuse; prevalence and service provision (a report on surveys and plans in English National Health Service regions).* London: Department of Health and Social Security, 1985.

22 Johnson AM. HIV and AIDS. *BMJ* 1991;**303**:573-6.

23 Department of Health and Social Security. *Guidelines of good clinical practice in the treatment of drug misusers.* London: HMSO, 1984.

24 Presidential Commission on the Human Immunodeficiency Virus Epidemic. *Watkins report.* Washington, DC: United States Government Printing Office, 1988.

25 Department of Health and Human Service. *Healthy people 2000.* Washington DC: DHHS, 1990.

26 Department of Health and Social Security. *Immunisation against infectious Disease.* London: HMSO, 1988.

27 Farrell M, Battersby M, Strang J. Screening for hepatitis B and vaccination of injecting drug users in NHS drug treatment services. *Br J Addict* 1990;**85**:1657-9.

28 Health Targets and Implementation (Health for All) Committee for Australian Health Ministers. *Health for all Australians.* Canberra: 1988:46-9.

29 Oppenheimer E, Sheehan M, Taylor C. Letting the client speak: drug misusers and the process of help-seeking. *Br J Addict* 1988;**83**:635-48.

30 Stimson GV, Alldritt L, Dolan K, Donoghoe M. Syringe exchange schemes for drug users in England and Scotland. *BMJ* 1988;**296**:1717-9.

31 Love J, Gossop M. The processes of referral and disposal within a London drug dependence clinic. *Br J Addict* 1986;**80**:435-40.

32 Dawe S, Griffiths P, Gossop M, Strang J. Should opiate addicts be involved in controlling their own detoxification? A comparison of fixed versus negotiable schedules. *Br J Addict* 1991;**86**:977-82.

33 Strang J. The roles of prescribing. In: Strang J, Stimson G, eds. *AIDS and drug misuse: the challenge for policy and practice in the 1990s.* London: Routledge, 1990.

34 Strang J, Heathcote S, Watson P. Habit-moderation in injecting drug addicts. *Health Trends* 1987;**19**:16-8.

35 McGlothlin WH, Anglin MD. Long-term follow-up of clients of high-dose and low-dose methadone programs. *Arch Gen Psychiatry* 1981;**38**:1055-63.

36 Ball JC, Lange WR, Myers CP, Friedman SR. Reducing the risk of AIDS through methadone maintenance treatment. *J Health Soc Behaviour* 1988; **29**:214-26.

37 Strang J, Marsh A, De Souza N. Hair analysis for drugs of abuse. *Lancet* 1990;**335**:740.

38 Home Office. *Tackling drug misuse: a summary of the government's strategy.* 2nd ed. London: HMSO, 1986.

39 Advisory Council on the Misuse of Drugs. *Report on treatment and rehabilitation.* London: HMSO, 1982.

40 Black D. Drug misuse: policy and service development. *J R Soc Health* 1988;**108**:83-9.

41 Strang J. Model service: turning the generalist on to drugs. In: MacGregor S, ed. *Drugs and British society: responses to a social problem in the 1980s.* London: Tavistock, 1989.

42 MacGregor S, Ettore B, Croomber R, Crosier A, Lodge H. *Drug services in England and the impact of the central funding initiative.* London: Insitute for the Study of Drug Dependence, 1990.

43 Strang J. Changing injecting practices; blunting the needle habit. *Br J Addict* 1988;**83**:237-9.

44 Scottish Committee on HIV infection and intravenous drug misuse. *Report on HIV infection in Scotland.* Edinburgh: Scottish Home and Health Department, 1986. (McClelland report.)

45 Strang J, Shah A. Notification of addicts and the medical practitioner: an evaluation of the system. *Br J Psychiatry* 1985;**147**:195-8.

46 Smart RG, Ogborne A. Losses to the addiction notification system. *Br J Addict* 1974;**69**:225-9.

47 Edwards G. The Home Office index as a basic monitoring system. In: Edwards G. Busch G, eds. *Drug problems in Britain; a review of ten years.* London: Academic Press, 1981:25-50.

48 Donmall M. Towards a national drug database. *Druglink* 1990;**5**:10-1.

209

Strategy full of good intentions

GAVIN MOONEY, ANDREW HEALEY

Previous chapters have examined several aspects of *The Health of the Nation*.[1] We shall look at the document from an economic perspective. We believe that the basis of the strategy set out in the green paper—establishing key areas and thereafter setting objectives and targets without ever considering cost—is seriously flawed.

From an economic perspective there are two criteria for judging the success or failure of a strategy such as that set out in *The Health of the Nation*: efficiency and equity. With respect to efficiency the key consideration is that as resources are always scarce it will never be possible to provide all the health for the nation that we would ideally like. We therefore have to choose which type of health or health care to pursue more and which to hold back on. The goal is to allocate the limited resources for improving health so as to maximise the benefit to society. With respect to equity, we simply note that *The Health of the Nation* says almost nothing.

The strategy

The document sets out suggested key areas which are determined on the basis of three criteria. Firstly, the area must constitute a big health problem; secondly, effective interventions must be available; and, thirdly, it should be possible to set objectives and targets. All three criteria must be met before the subject is judged to be a key area.

What is far from clear is how these three criteria are used to arrive at the choice of the key areas. There is virtually no quantification of the extent to which interventions will be effective—just some hope that targets can be achieved. The difficulty with this approach is simply explained. Intervention in a big problem may need to have only a low effectiveness to do much good in terms of health gains. Similarly, highly effective intervention in a small problem may still do as much good, as is the case with chiropody.[2] The document does not make it clear how these factors have been brought together to judge what combination of investment in different areas provides the greatest effectiveness in terms of health gains.

There is also the difficulty that in defining the size of a problem there are two dimensions: premature death and avoidable ill health. The document gives no indication of the relative weight to be attached to these dimensions. A third problem is that if objectives and targets cannot be set for a particular area that debars it from being designated a key area and thereby prevents it from being given high priority.

What is of more fundamental concern, however, is that the costs of implementation are not considered in deciding on a key area or what the target should be. Thus if an area presents a big health problem, has effective interventions, and is targetable, whether the interventions are expensive is deemed irrelevant. That seems particularly bad logic when resources are scarce.

An alternative

Fortunately there is an alternative and it is simple. A successful strategy must consider the size of problem together with the potential quantified impact of interventions so that a benefit is estimated; must use some weighting to identify the relative importances of saving life and reducing morbidity; must take costs of interventions into account; and must weigh up use of resources in one way against their use in other competing areas. Key areas should be selected on the basis that more resources are better spent there than elsewhere or that more resources are better spent there even at the expense of reducing the resources for another area.

This last point is one that the document signally fails to pick up, indeed passes over rather glibly. Thus in the foreword William Waldegrave states: "It must be right to redouble our efforts to reduce avoidable disease and premature death. This must not, however, be at the expense of caring for ill people. . . ."

Our proposal overcomes all the problems we have highlighted above. If more resources are to be spent on health then we need an

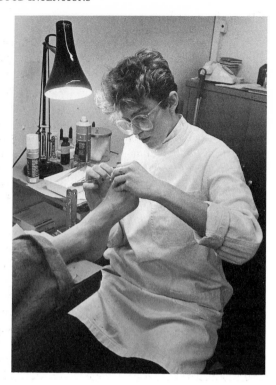

Effective intervention in
a small problem can
produce large health
gains

indicator that allows us to assess the effectiveness of using them in one
area compared with that in another. Though measuring health status
—for example, through quality adjusted life years (QALYs)—is not
yet an exact science and indeed never will be,[3] at least many health
status measures address the right issue in that they bring together
mortality and morbidity in a single index. We suggest that measures
of health be combined with information on costing to allow "marginal
cost per QALY" to be assessed—for example, if we spend £x more
how many QALYs do we get from intervening on this problem and
how many from intervening on another problem? And where extra
resources can buy most QALYs that is where the resources should be
allocated.[4]

This simple approach to a health strategy would allow the health of
the nation to be improved to the greatest extent whatever resources
are available.[5] Yet the strategy document fails to get even close to such
an approach. As a result it is flawed in its central logic.

212

Objectives and targets

A large part of the document is concerned with the objectives for the chosen key areas and what the quantified targets are. With respect to the objectives we suggest that there is a case for re-examining these often rather vague statements to see whether they represent the true objectives of the population. For example, the objective for the cancer programme is stated as, "To reduce death and ill-health from cancers." However, the emphasis is on screening for breast cancer and cervical cancer. Although whether the emphasis is justified is debatable, what is more important is to recognise the concept of reassurance or avoidance of anxiety in such screening programmes. For these health services and many others there is more to the objectives than just health.[6]

The targets given in the green paper are in practise quantification of the objectives. The target for coronary heart disease, for example, is a 30% reduction nationally in death in people aged under 65 years. Why 30%? Why not 40% or 28%? The basis for many of the targets seems to be: "This is where we are heading according to current trends. So if we set the target just a bit better than that, then maybe we can present the challenge to get there." That is a rather appealing way of looking at the issue, but we would question whether it is a sensible way of planning the health of a nation. If the target were set at 28% for deaths from coronary heart disease, what would the implications be for use of resources? And if it were 40%—would it mean that far too many resources were spent on coronary heart disease in the sense that the loss of opportunity would be too high in other programmes? These key issues are not even raised, far less answered, in the strategy document.

Thus the targets are not based on efficiency concerns and consequently are most unlikely to promote efficient use of resources in the future health strategy. The good intentions on which the document is based are admirable. The question is whether they are an adequate basis for promoting the health of the nation.

1 Secretary of State for Health. *The health of the nation.* London: HMSO, 1991. (Cm 1523.)
2 Bryan S, Parkin D, Donaldson C. Chiropody and the QALY: a case study in assigning disability and distress to patients. *Health Policy* 1991;**18**:169-85.
3 Loomes G, McKenzie L. The use of QALYs in health care decision making. *Soc Sci Med* 1989;**28**:299-308.
4 Williams A. The economics of coronary artery bypass grafting. *BMJ* 1985;**291**:326-9.
5 Donaldson C, Mooney G. Needs assessment, priority setting, and contracts: an economic perspective. *BMJ* (in press).
6 McGuire A, Henderson J, Mooney G. *The economics of health care. An introductory text.* London:

What the government should do

SHEILA ADAM, SPENCER HAGARD

In his foreword to *The Health of the Nation* the secretary of state throws down a gauntlet not only to the NHS but also to Whitehall. He reminds ministers and politicians, as well as the NHS and the people it serves, that it is the responsibility of his office to "take all such steps as may be desirable to secure the preparation, effective carrying out and coordination of measures conducive to the health of the people."[1]

The challenges are immense. How to ensure that the NHS uses its finite resources to provide services that are clinically effective, appropriate for each patient's needs, responsive to user preferences, and value for money. How to jolt other central government departments out of their constitutionally established sectional interests and into a commitment to better health. And how to set the process in a framework which is genuinely democratic and participatory and thus more likely to deliver better health.

Can *The Health of the Nation* offer the first step towards a comprehensive health strategy for England? We believe that it can, but only if the government is prepared to recognise and respond to the criticisms of the document and then establish a long term planning and implementation strategy. It must also take steps to ensure early integration of the strategy into both NHS and multisectoral activities.

The criticisms

Criticism of *The Health of the Nation* is becoming an industry, with critics coming from all sides. We have summarised what we consider

214

to be five key criticisms and indicated the ways we think the government should respond.

Although the document describes progress on the World Health Organisation European region 38 targets, the approach has been criticised for failing to encompass the WHO global strategy for Health for All initiated in 1977,[2] and for not building on international experience in developing local Health for All strategies (which have been summarised in a publication from the Department of Health's operational research service.[3] Thus, *The Health of the Nation* does not, for example, refer to the essential prerequisites for achieving the health targets: peace and freedom from fear of war, equal opportunities for all, and the satisfaction of basic needs (adequate food and income, basic education, safe water and sanitation, decent housing, secure work, and a satisfying role in society). Sceptics, many of whom are highly committed to the concept of a health strategy, have described the government's approach as too narrow and overmedicalised.

In particular the document has been criticised for failing to deal with strategic issues relating to inequalities. Equity and participation are stressed in Health for All strategies but not in *The Health of the Nation*. Health inequalities are real and associated primarily with income, social networks and perceived social worth, and lifestyle.[4] The variables are linked but each also operates independently.

The next criticism has been expressed in two opposite directions. Firstly, that the strategy focuses too much on the NHS and, secondly, that it focuses too much on other sectors. The temptation to interpret equal noise on both sides as a positive sign should be resisted as an effective strategy needs to balance both elements. There are clear opportunities for the NHS to use its resources more effectively to achieve health gain, but it can have only limited impact on wider health problems.

Harsher critics have described *The Health of the Nation* as little more than pre-election political flannel, though this was not the view of the shadow health secretary Robin Cook; he welcomed the initiative. But critics point out that even if the Department of Health is seriously committed to it, the lack of commitment and priority from other departments may be too powerful for the Secretary of State for Health to overcome.

The priority areas have also been criticised: the inclusions, the exclusions, and the specific targets. Previous articles have commented in detail and we will add only two comments. Firstly, the danger of

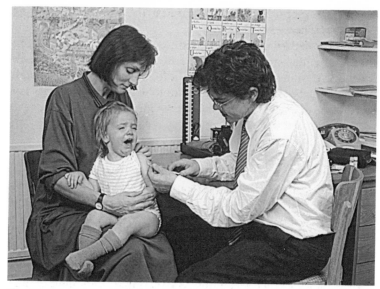

Corporate contracts must include more health targets such as that for childhood immunisation

considering only the easily measurable. As McLellan's article on rehabilitation showed,[5] even the harder to measure can be included and hardening the softer targets in priority areas needs to be an early research and development priority. Secondly, the exclusion of elderly people and their needs, both explicitly in the absence of a separate section in the green paper and implicitly in the emphasis on premature mortality, must be remedied in the white paper.

Government's response to criticism

The government must signal that it has heard and is prepared to respond to criticisms of *The Health of the Nation*, and the white paper should provide for:

● Closer alignment with Health for All by the Year 2000 and a determination to learn from the experience of other countries
● A crossdepartmental approach (at central government level) to health and social policy that relates health and social gain to wealth creation and use of resources
● Additional resources to develop and implement a health strategy. These should include bridging funds to enable new areas of work to

begin in advance of resources being released from activities that will no longer be necessary
● Action to address problems such as low income, poor housing, unemployment, and subsidies on unhealthy food, all of which are known to have an adverse effect on health. Initially the action is likely to be limited, but the government needs to begin to move to a position in which all of its policies are consistent with its health strategy.

Short term strategies: the next three years

The immediate priority is to create acceptance and gain time for the full development of the health strategy and construction of all the necessary means to assure its implementation. The green paper is ambitious and has raised many legitimate aspirations. It is particularly at risk in a pre-election period. The proposed strategy represents a major reorientation of health policy and implies a considerable reorientation of other sectors of society. Time, commitment, and considerable human effort will be needed to plan and implement its long term success. The government's most urgent responsibilities are therefore to begin a programme of work to ensure robust implementation, and, at the same time, to ensure that some early results are achieved which can assist its acceptance.

The NHS Management Executive holds regional health authorities to account, and these authorities similarly hold their constituent district health authorities and family health services authorities to account through individual corporate contracts. These represent the range of key objectives that each authority agrees to achieve by a defined date. Initially, the focus of corporate contracts has been on finance, activity, and manpower, but during 1991-2 corporate contracts have often included objectives on immunisation, breast and cervical screening, and other outcome related issues such as resettlement programmes for long stay hospital residents with mental illness or learning difficulties.

Although these objectives apply to only limited areas and are measured by process rather than outcome, they represent an initial attempt to build health targets into the management framework. With the publication of the green paper and associated changes following the NHS reforms, the management executive must follow up its guidance for 1992-3[6] and strengthen the health target component of the corporate contract. Given the continuing central priority given to

217

financial control,[7] these changes will require considerable determination and courage in Whitehall.

The corporate contract represents an amalgam of central direction and local priorities. The health strategy, while requiring clear government leadership, must also reflect the views and preferences of local communities. Assessment of needs is not simply a technical issue with "right" answers. Rather it must incorporate values and preferences alongside epidemiological, clinical, and technical advice. For example, the professional advice on the relative needs for neonatal intensive care and for services for mentally frail people can help decision making but must be considered in the context of the preferences and priorities of the local community.

It will therefore be necessary to require health authorities to defend publicly the basis of their health priorities. Various approaches are available—for example, surveys (self completed or by interview), open meetings, panels as in market research methods, or community participative approaches using existing groups and opinion leaders. For most health authorities this is a new activity and there are no tried and tested methods. A dialogue between health authorities and their residents will, however, be essential if the national direction of health targets is to be balanced by a rounded view of local needs and priorities. To assure success, a health strategy must be seen to be founded on the principles of democracy and citizenry; the experiences of formulating Healthy People 1990 and Healthy People 2000 in the United States provide confirmatory evidence.[8]

Health targets require the NHS to do things better and other sections of society to become fully committed to health. Two major strands of change management therefore need to be created and woven together. There is a risk of losing the symmetry, either through clinicians or NHS managers, or both, failing to contribute to the wider social agenda or through the issues being regarded by politicians as exclusively within the NHS. Two examples relating to suggested health priorities illustrate this.

The first example relates to coronary heart disease. The NHS is responsible for diagnosing and treating this disease and at least some of its risk factors and each year spends £500m on these activities.[9] Clinicians and managers need to ensure that the available resources are used to maximum effect—that procedures are introduced only after proper evaluation, that services reflect the wishes of their users, and that the care provided for each patient is appropriate for his or her needs. If these principles are followed benefits will ensue and will almost certainly include release of some resources as well as better quality care.

The second example relates to smoking, the single most important preventable cause of death and ill health. Creating a positive climate of public opinion, developing health education in schools, and the increased role of general practitioners in helping smokers to stop, have all contributed to a decrease in smoking over the past 20 years, especially among non-manual workers and their families. Smoking rates among manual workers remain higher and the fall among women has been substantially less than among men. A recent study showed no decrease in smoking prevalence among schoolchildren.[10] The commitment of clinicians to a national health strategy will depend on ministers ensuring that effective action is taken in other sectors to support the NHS in reducing smoking prevalence. The continuing failure of government to outlaw the advertising and promotion of tobacco threatens its credibility with clinicians and their commitment to the strategy.

Credibility with managers will be determined by the priority government is prepared to maintain for *The Health of the Nation.* Health service managers have delivered a major change agenda coupled with considerable reductions in resources over the past three years. There is evidence that at least a significant minority are enthused by the health gain agenda. But there is a limit to the hours in the day and, if the government really wants health targets achieved it may have to be prepared to make slower progress on some other important issues.

Finally, the strategy for health will need to exert a major influence on the new agenda for research and development in the NHS[11]; this implies the government standing firm against the research and development programme being dominated by biomedical scientists or even clinical scientists. Instead it must be focused on enabling the NHS to improve health both directly, through its own sphere of action, and indirectly, through its influence on other organisations. Research will therefore need to be related to policy development and implementation, to enable the programme to enhance decision making throughout the NHS and other sectors.

Longer term strategies: the next 43 years

A national strategy for health, once developed, needs to continue forever, and therefore a useful vantage point from which to consider the construction of longer term strategies is the year 2034, which lies as far in the future as the foundation of the NHS does in our past. A strong health policy is most likely to be reached if a health strategy is firmly established in the first full parliament of the first British health strategy. The first strategy should include the following measures.

Firstly, a broad political and social consensus needs to be achieved not only for the concept of a national health strategy (a situation which now seems close) but for the necessary innovations in policy making and implementation which will be required to nurture and sustain it. These innovations are by no means assured; indeed the need for them has been largely ignored in the national strategy debate so far. The changes needed are:

- Charging the Secretary of State for Health with explicit responsibility for coordinating and monitoring the efforts to achieve the national strategy in all sectors of society—both other government departments (directly at national level) and the remainder of society (through the NHS authorities at national, regional, and local levels)
- Providing the resources at all levels to take the strategy forward and implement it. This is currently the most underdiscussed issue of all. We are not used to working across sectors in our society and have tended to attribute past failures (for example, in joint health and local authority planning) to anything but its root cause of insufficient intellectual and managerial investment. We seem unaware of the great development effort which will be needed to implement a national health strategy.

Secondly, NHS management needs to be harnessed more securely to measures necessary to achieve health gain—for example, applying sound management to existing knowledge, as in subjects such as managing cervical screening programmes and preventing stroke, and cost effectiveness in research investment, such as in measures to support greater contentment among infirm elderly people or higher levels of physical activity in the population.

Thirdly, investment in surveillance, analysis, and assessment should be increased to greatly improve recognition of health problems and analysis of determinants; identification of the potential for specific improvements in health; identification of the specific knowledge we require; and consequent information gathering and research. Lastly, all these measures should be undertaken in collaborative programmes with other nations which are drawing up national health strategies.

Conclusions

Although we recognise the validity of many of the criticisms of *The Health of the Nation*, we warmly welcome its publication. If the government responds positively we believe that a framework can be established which will ensure the better health of our population.

As Smith said in a recent paper,[12] health can be viewed in two ways:

Individuals are healthy to the extent that their mental and physical capabilities permit them to discharge the obligations and enjoy the rewards associated with membership of their community, while that community is healthy to the extent that its members are healthy in this sense.

This definition implies two distinct but complementary strategies for the pursuit of improved public health: one aims to promote the capabilities of individuals so that they may function in the widest diversity of social contexts; the other aims to promote such a diversity of social contexts as to permit successful functioning for individuals with the widest diversity of capabilities. We have made some progress with the first kind of strategy but have scarcely begun to embark on the second.

With government vision, commitment, and resolution, the health strategy could enable us for the first time to address these two complementary approaches to securing the better health of our population.

1 Secretary of State for Health. *The health of the nation*. London: HMSO, 1991. (Cm 1523.)
2 World Health Organisation. *Thirtieth world health assembly resolution WHA 30. 43*. Geneva: WHO, 1977.
3 Barnes R. *Setting strategic health goals: experience in other couuntries*. London: Department of Health Operational Research Service, 1990.
4 Blaxter M. *Health and lifestyles* London: Tavistock Routledge, 1990.
5 McLellan DL. Rehabilitation. *BMJ* 1991;**303**:355-7.
6 Department of Health. *Priorities and planning guidance for the NHS for 1992/93*. London: DoH, 1991. (EL(91)103.)
7 House of Commons Select Committee on Health. *Public expenditure on health and social services. Third report from the health committee: session 1990/91*. Vol 1. London: HMSO, 1991. (Paper 614.)
8 Sullivan LW. Foreward, In: *Healthy people 2000*. Washington, DC: Department of Health and Human Services, 1990.
9 Health Education Authority. *Health update 1: coronary heart disease*. London: HEA, 1990.
10 Social Survey Division, Office of Population Censuses and Surveys. *Smoking among secondary school children in 1990*. London: HMSO, 1991.
11 Department of health. *Research for health: a research and development strategy for the NHS*. London: HMSO, 1991.
12 Smith A. *A national health service and the public health*. Harrogate: Yorkshire Regional Health Authority, 1991.

Letters to the Editor, *BMJ*

While the series, "The Health of the Nation: responses," was running in the "BMJ", the Editor invited readers to contribute to the debate through the correspondence columns of the Journal. Published below are some of the letters received up to the time of going to press.

Sir,—The Radical Statistics Health Group has pointed out the lack of a strategy for health of the nation; many critics have focused and will continue to focus on the lack of attention in the document to social inequalities as a reason for ill health. Such criticism seems to me to miss the point. It is poor social conditions, not inequality, that cause poor health. If the poorest in the country lived in decent housing, had jobs that gave them an adequate income and self respect, did not smoke, did not drink alcohol to excess, had an adequate diet, and took enough physical exercise it would not matter at all whether the richest lived in more or less similar circumstances or were immensely better off.

The consequence of this line of argument is that we need a strategy that ensures the poorest have what they need to be healthy. We also need more information (though we already have quite a bit) concerning the social conditions and lifestyles that are, in fact, necessary for health. The lack of attention in *The Health of the Nation* to altering environmental circumstances is deplorable and means that it is unlikely that meaningful targets can be set or met in the fields of childhood asthma and childhood accidents and in conditions related to lifestyle, such as coronary heart disease. But this is not because too little attention is given to the irrelevant concept of inequality.

PHILIP GRAHAM

Department of Child Psychiatry,
Hospital for Sick Children,
Great Ormond Street,
London WC1N 3JH

1 Radical Statistics Health Group. Missing: a strategy for health of the nation. *BMJ* 1991;**303**:299-302. (3 August.)

Sir,—The Health of the Nation series has got off to an unfortunate start. The first article, by the Radical Health Statistics Group, presents such a negative, biased, and distorted picture of the consultation document that one could almost accuse the group of being party political.[1] Anyone reading the paper would indeed be left with the impression that "all the components necessary for a national programme aimed at enhancing the nation's health are absent"; that the question of inequalities in health had been totally overlooked; and that the requirement to find new ways of measuring improvements in health had been omitted.

It seems only fair to point out that the authors of this article have deliberately ignored the paragraphs in the green paper which describe the need for government "to take effective action on behalf of individuals and their families"; identify how progress in addressing inequalities in health could be made; and outline a varied programme of research and development to support better monitoring of health in the future.[2]

By accusing the government of confusing a strategy for health with a strategy for the health service, it is clear that they themselves are confused. In claiming that the scope for improving health largely lies outside the NHS, they clearly do not understand that "health" is a multidimensional concept which includes, for example, enjoyment as well as duration of life; freedom from pain as well as relief from discomfort. They obviously have not registered, either, the growing responsibilities of health authorities to purchase a range of NHS and non-NHS services which achieve better health and to develop local health strategies with other agencies.

Some of the arguments which they use, supported by references,[3-5] are no more than a collection of value judgments or half truths. Furthermore, no real solutions are put forward as alternatives to the many issues which are raised. Those of us "who have a heart to help" and not just censure the government's proposals for a national strategy for health will recognise the ease with which sneers or yawns can kill off new initiatives such as these.

Let us hope that the rest of the series will offer practical and constructive suggestions on what might be included in a future white paper and thereby make a genuine contribution to this important debate.

JACKY CHAMBERS

Health Education Authority,
London WC1H 9TX

1 Radical Health Statistics Group. Missing in a strategy for health of the nation. *BMJ* 1991;**303**:299-302. (3 August.)
2 Secretary of State for Health. *The health of the nation*. London: HMSO, 1991:v,ix, 19,20;ch 7.
3 Health Education Authority. *National opinion poll consumer health education survey 1987-89*. London: HEA, 1991.
4 Health Education Authority. *Heart disease in the 1990s. A strategy for 1990-95*. London: HEA, 1989. (Health Education Authority Look After Your Heart programme.)
5 Wilkinson RG. Income distribution and mortality. *Sociology of Health and Illness* 1990;**12**:391-412.

SIR,—Dr S Bingham's response to *The Health of the Nation* discusses the role of government in food policy.[1] There is another area in which the government is able to influence food policy at no additional cost. The Common Agricultural Policy (CAP) now consumes over 30bn European currency units annually[2] (£1=1·43 ecus); much of this is spent in subsidising unhealthy foods. Two examples involving saturated fats are the payment on the butterfat content of milk and a minimum fat content for the top prices on animal carcasses. A third example is the subsidy on tobacco growing.

We are encouraged to drink skimmed milk and to trim excess fat off meat. It would be more efficient, and improve the nation's diet, if there was no incentive to produce excess saturated fat. If we are going to subsidise food production then the policy should also aim to improve health.

KEITH NEAL

Sheffield Health Authority,
Sheffield S11 8EU

1 Bingham S. Dietary aspects of a health strategy for England. *BMJ* 1991;**303**:353-5. (10 August.)
2 Against the grain. *The Economist* 1991 July 6-12:48-9.

SIR,—Dr Jacky Chambers's letter[1] attacking our response[2] to *The Health of the Nation*[3] is bedevilled by the confusion of which she accuses us but gives us an opportunity to clarify our political position and reinforce some points that we made in our article.

Our name is Radical Statistics Health Group, not Radical Health Statistics Group, as in Dr Chambers's letter. Her suggestion that "one could almost accuse the group of being party political" is untrue. Radical Statistics, of which we are part, has never been affiliated to any political party or other organisation apart from the now defunct British Society for Social Responsibility in Science. Our first publications criticised misleading use of statistics in documents produced by the last Labour government.[4 5] Since 1979 we have criticised misuse of statistics by Conservative governments.[6 7] We will continue to criticise any political party that uses statistics misleadingly in government or in opposition, irrespective of whether people within our group support its political aims.

On the other hand, the view that statistics is a branch of political science is not new. It was held by the social and sanitary reformers who in the 1830s founded the Statistical Society of London, later to become the Royal Statistical Society. Their aim of "ascertaining and bringing together of those 'facts which are calculated to illustrate the condition and prospects of society' . . . with the view to determine those principles on which the well-being of society depends"[8] contrasts with the narrow focus on "individuals and their families" that underpins current political policy in general and the green paper in particular.

Our critique of the green paper arose from a dissatisfaction with the avalanche of articles written by people who, in their enthusiasm to welcome an opportunity for health promotion, failed to balance this with a critical analysis of what *The Health of the Nation* actually contained. We could not on this occasion put forward positive alternatives and this was not in the brief given to us by the *BMJ*, and we knew that a further 20 articles had been commissioned to do just that. We are interested in alternative approaches, and these were on the agenda of the conference that we held on 21 September jointly with the Public Health Alliance.

We reject Dr Chambers's allegation that we "do not understand that 'health' is a multidimensional concept." A rereading will show that this was made explicit in our article and that we pointed to the need for action outside the NHS. This action should go beyond the limited range of activity proposed and cannot be achieved simply, as Dr Chambers suggests, by health authorities purchasing "a range of NHS and non-NHS services."[1] Far from ignoring the sections of the green paper that referred briefly to inequalities in health and the need for better data, we pointed out that they were not prominently placed in the document and did not explore the problems in any depth. We are mystified by Dr Chambers's accusation that our arguments, supported by references, "are no more than a collection of value judgments or half truths" and find it strange that of the three of our 49 references that she cites to support this view, two come from her own organisation.

Our critique of *The Health of the Nation* is not a dismissal of the need to promote health but an analysis of its lack of proposals for "effective action." Dr Chambers suggests that this should not deter those "who have a heart to help" from putting their weight behind it. We are unconvinced. As statisticians, epidemiologists, and public health doctors we do not hesitate to criticise suggestions from clinicians that, in the absence of effective remedies, ineffective or unproved remedies should be applied. So why should we tolerate this in our own specialty of public health?

RADICAL STATISTICS HEALTH GROUP

1 Chambers J. The health of the nation. *BMJ* 1991;**303**:520. (31 August.)
2 Radical Statistics Health Group. Missing: a strategy for the health of the nation. *BMJ* 1991;**303**:299-302. (3 August.)
3 Department of Health. *The health of the nation.* London: HMSO, 1991.
4 Radical Statistics Health Group. *Whose priorities? A critique of "Priorities for Health and Personal Social Services in England."* London: Radical Statistics, 1976.
5 Radical Statistics Health Group. *RAW(P) deals. A critique of "Sharing resources for health in England."* London: Radical Statistics, 1977.
6 Radical Statistics Health Group. *Unsafe in their hands.* London: Radical Statistics, 1985.
7 Radical Statistics Health Group. *Facing the figures: what really is happening to the National Health Service?* London: Radical Statistics, 1987.
8 Introduction. *Journal of the Statistical Society of London.* 1839;I:1-5.

SIR,—It is encouraging that *The Health of the Nation* recognises rehabilitation as an area in which there is clear scope for improvement.[1] It also recognises the importance of multisectoral influences: "health is determined by a wide range of influences from . . . family and social circumstances to the physical and social environment."

As someone with a disability, I find this the right sort of talk. People with disabilities have on average lower incomes than the rest of the population.[2] Many buildings, leisure facilities, and public transport are inaccessible.[3] Two thirds of disabled people aged under 65 are unemployed.[2] Much support at home is inadequate, and there is a shortage of appropriate housing. Improvements in these aspects have the potential to improve health much more than medical services alone. Though medical services offering rehabilitation should not be neglected and there are things to be welcomed in the green paper, the concern for a multisectoral approach does not extend to disability.

Professor D L McLellan begins to touch on this by setting targets such as increasing employment and by recognising that work with social services, housing, etc, is required.[4] It is to be hoped that this is built into the consultation. To improve the lot of disabled people, however, the wider dimensions of health need more emphasis. Especially at national level, where the aim should be to effect multisectoral change, policies are required across departments, coordinating legislation. Targets might include reducing the number of people in residential accommodation against their will by 75% (in coordination with community care policies and local authorities); ensuring that all public transport is accessible; increasing the proportion of disabled people in employment, as Professor McLellan suggested[4]; introducing legislation against discrimination, making it impossible to discriminate against the disabled in employment, for example; and alleviating poverty among the disabled (perhaps with a disability income). Above all, the approach must encompass the realisation that disability is not about people with problems but about a society that can't or won't adapt to a substantial minority.

Pie in the sky? It shouldn't be if as a society we believe that people with disabilities ought to be treated as equals.

IAN BASNETT

London E1 9BE

1 Secretary of State for Health. *The health of the nation*, London: HMSO, 1991. (Cm 1523.)
2 Martin J, White A. *The financial circumstances of disabled adults living in private households*. London: HMSO, 1988. (Office of Population Censuses and Surveys report 2.)
3 Greater London Association for the Disabled. *A consumer study of public transport handicap in Greater London*. London: GLAD, 1986.
4 McLellan DL. Rehabilitation. *BMJ* 1991;**303**:355-7. (10 August.)

SIR,—In common with others we have been considering our response to the government's paper *The Health of the Nation*.[1] As part of this process we have looked at the applicability, at district health authority level, of the document's suggested mortality targets.

Because of the very small numbers involved, problems of interpretation of infant mortality trends at district health authority level have long been recognised; there is, however, a temptation to assume that the greater number of deaths in adults at district level, at least for the major causes, make chance variation less likely and so make the analysis of mortality trends statistically robust. If true this would facilitate the direct translation of the mortality targets suggested in *The Health of the Nation* into district targets. Although not explicitly recommended in the government's paper, this approach to measuring changes in health is appealing because such district based data are routinely available.

Nevertheless, calculating the mortality trends for the major causes of adult death in our own health authority has shown that, even though the numerator for the rates may be larger than for infant mortality, the denominator is also increased. The effect of this is to again render even quite large percentage changes in mortality over time liable to chance variation. For example, there was an apparent decrease of 12·1% in deaths from coronary heart disease from 1981 to 1989 for men aged 35-64 in Hull. However, the 95% confidence intervals for this change in mortality are wide ($-2·7\times10^{-4}$ to $1·2\times10^{-3}$) and allow the possibility either of no change or of an increase in the true mortality for men of this age. Indeed, the same uncertainty is true of the district mortality trends for all the conditions suggested in *The Health of the Nation*.

We suggest, therefore, that changes in death rates are a statistically inappropriate method of measuring variations over time in the health of a district population. This is a further argument for the need to develop measures of health that are not based on mortality for use at district level.

SUE IBBOTSON
IAN WATT

Department of Public Health Medicine,
Hull Health Authority,
Hull HU2 8TD

1 Secretary of State for Health. *The health of the nation.* London: HMSO, 1991.

SIR,—Dr S Bingham, in her article on dietary aspects of a health strategy for England, recognises that health education on its own is insufficient as a policy for dietary change.[1] National food culture, food advertising, and nutrition labelling are appropriately highlighted as areas in need of public attention. The green paper and Dr Bingham's response to it neglect the crucial economic dimensions of personal income, food prices, and fiscal policy in agriculture.

Low income is an obstacle to healthy eating. The Department of Health's recent dietary survey shows that those in receipt of welfare benefits have comparatively low intakes of vitamins C, D, and E as well as calcium and magnesium.[2] Foods providing dietary fibre and micronutrients, such as oranges and wholemeal bread, are expensive sources of food energy. For example, two custard cream biscuits at 3p and 1 lb of carrots at 20p each provides 0·42 MJ.[3] Healthy eating is a luxury for the increasing number of those below or on the margins of poverty in Britain. In 1988, 11·8 million people, including 25% of the nation's children, were dependent on incomes of less than 50% of the average wage.[4] Financial hardship tends also to limit access to food. Those without a car may not be able to reach good supermarkets or to shop cheaply in bulk.[3] Those without a well equipped kitchen are unable to store and prepare food in the most appropriate ways.[3] There is therefore certainly a case for reviewing current levels of welfare benefit to make a healthy diet at least potentially accessible for the whole nation.[5]

E J BRUNNER

Department of Community Medicine,
University College London,
London WC1E 6EA

1 Bingham S. Dietary aspects of a health strategy for England. *BMJ* 1991;**303**:353-5. (10 August.)
2 Gregory J, Foster K, Tyler H, Wiseman M. *The dietary and nutritional survey of British adults.* London: HMSO, 1990.
3 Cole-Hamilton I, Lobstein TJ. *Poverty and nutrition survey.* London: National Children's Homes, 1991.

4 House of Commons Social Security Committee. *Low income statistics: households below average income*. London: HMSO, 1991.
5 Radical Statistics Health Group. *Facing the figures*. London: Radical Statistics, 1987.

SIR,—Professor I B Pless's comments on accident prevention in his response to *The Health of the Nation* should be noted by politicians, officials in the Department of Health, and all health workers.[1] What he is asking is for the Department of Health to take a firm lead in accident prevention (injury control in North American terminology). The justification for this is sound. Accidents are the leading cause of death in the early years of life. In the United States they account for a greater proportion of years of potential life lost than cancer and heart disease combined. They cause much suffering and hardship. They lose the NHS millions of pounds a year.

In supporting Professor Pless's proposals for a division of injury control in the Department of Health I would go even further. I believe that until the discipline is given a similar status to heart disease, cancer, and communicable disease control it will not make any real progress.

For advances to be made an institute (or centre) for accident prevention and injury control attached to an academic institution in the United Kingdom is urgently needed. Such an institute would have a similar role to that of the Communicable Diseases Surveillance Centre. It would act as a clearing house for information on accidents but also collate and stimulate research. It would act as a national focus for action on accidents.

Some will argue that such an institute already exists in the form of the Medical Commission on Accident Prevention, the Child Accident Prevention Trust, and the Parliamentary Advisory Council on Transport Safety (PACTS). These important organisations are either too specialised or too restricted within their terms of reference. The Royal Society for the Prevention of Accidents operates on a broader front, especially in education. It has already taken a considerable initiative towards working more closely with health authorities with the production of its report *Action on Accidents* in conjunction with the National Association of Health Authorities and Trusts.[2] Despite all this activity the need for a national institute still exists.

Several regional and district health authorities have now developed strategies and plans for accident prevention. They cannot go it alone. The government must play its part. As no other agency is likely to take the lead the Department of Health should seize the initiative, recognise its key role, and put substantial resources into making appreciable inroads into this major modern epidemic.

JAMES GORDON AVERY

Flecknoe,
Near Rugby,
Warwickshire CV23 8AT

1 Pless IB. Accident prevention. *BMJ* 1991;**303**:462-4.
2 National Association of Health Authorities and Royal Society for the Prevention of Accidents Strategy Group. *Report. Action on accidents: the unique role of the health service*. Birmingham: NAHA, 1990.

SIR,—Drs Martin Dennis and Charles Warlow's proposed strategy for stroke[1] in response to *The Health of the Nation* ignores the potentially large contribution of oestrogen replacement treatment in preventing stroke in postmenopausal women: it is estimated to reduce the relative risk by about half in this group.[2] Reductions in the relative risks of killing or disabling diseases that have been reported in controlled studies of oestrogen replacement treatment with or without balancing progestogens include for strokes 0·53,[2] myocardial infarction 0·30,[3] and hip fracture 0·33.[4] Additionally, there are significant reductions in other fractures related to osteoporosis.[5 6]

These observations are supported by a decreased mortality in women using oestrogen replacement treatment.[7] In the absence of circulating oestrogens there is a threefold to fourfold increase in atherosclerosis in postmenopausal women.[8] With one exception,[9] these figures for the reduction of relative risks have been confirmed to various degrees by other studies.

Oestrogen replacement treatment should be considered in calculations of strategies for decreasing the risk of stroke and improving the health of the nation.

ALLAN ST J DIXON

Chairman,
National Osteoporosis Society,
PO Box 10,
Radstock,
Bath BA3 3YB

1 Dennis M, Warlow C. Strategy for stroke. *BMJ* 1991;**303**:636-8. (14 September.)
2 Paganini-Hill A, Ross RK, Henderson BE. Postmenopausal oestrogen treatment and stroke: a prospective study. *BMJ* 1988;**297**:519-22.
3 Stampfer MJ, Willet WC, Colditz GA, Rosner B, Speizer FE, Hennekens CA. A prospective study of estrogen therapy and coronary heart disease. *N Engl J Med* 1985;**313**:1044-9.
4 Kiel DP, Felson DT, Anderson JJ, Wilson PW, Moskewitz MA. Hip fractures and the use of estrogens in postmenopausal women, the Framingham study. *N Engl J Med* 1987;**317**: 1169-74.
5 Lindsay R, Hart DM, Forrest C, Baird C. Prevention of spinal osteoporosis in oophorectomised women. *Lancet* 1980;ii: 1152-4.
6 Hutchinson TA, Polansky SM, Feinstein AR. Postmenopausal oestrogens protect against fractures of hip and distal radius, a case control study. *Lancet* 1979;ii: 705-9.
7 Henderson BE, Paganini-Hill A, Ross RK. Decreased mortality in users of estrogen replacement therapy. *Arch Intern Med* 1991;**151**:75-8.
8 Witteman JCM, Grobbee DE, Kok FJ, Hofman A, Valkenburg HA. Increased risk of atherosclerosis in women after the menopause. *BMJ* 1989;**289**:642-4.
9 Wilson PWF, Garrison RJ, Castelli WP. Postmenopausal estrogen use, cigarette smoking and cardiovascular morbidity in women over 50. *N Engl J Med* 1985;**313**:1038-43.

SIR,—We should like to emphasise some of the important points in Dr P G J Burney's article on a strategy for asthma,[1] points that are in danger of being lost in the epidemiological arguments.

It is essential to include asthma as a key area because it is the commonest chronic disease affecting all age groups in England, and because it is a major cause of preventable deaths and ill health; it is the only cause of preventable death with a higher standardised mortality ratio in 1987 than in 1979.

The consultative document and Dr Burney have accepted this necessity, but both imply controversy as to whether intervention reduces suffering and whether targets may be set. Repeated studies have shown that there are preventable factors in over 80% of deaths.[2] One study showed that if patients with severe asthma were admitted under a general medical firm they were 10 times more likely to be readmitted than if their initial care had been under a respiratory physician.[3] Suffering results from underuse of regular preventive treatments, and yet these reduce symptoms,[4] may reduce risk of the airway narrowing becoming fixed,[5] and are more effective than relieving broncho-dilator treatments.[6] They have also been shown to reduce school absenteeism due to asthma.[7]

The current debate about treatment with β agonists and possible side effects of inhaled steroids should not be allowed to imply that there is no consensus on how to treat asthma. In perhaps no other condition has there been such clear agreement as to management of both children[8] and adults.[9 10] In adults the recommended shift away from dependence on regular treatment with β agonists, and the recommendations regarding reducing absorption of inhaled steroids, predated the subsequent controversies and are not influenced by them.

We accept the argument that in setting targets allowances must be made for the increasing prevalence of the condition. We also recognise that high rates of admission to hospital due to asthma may be a good, rather than a bad, phenomenon. Nevertheless, as 80% of deaths involve preventable factors we must set a target for their future reduction and establish now a confidential inquiry into these deaths. There should also be a target for a greater proportion of patients in hospital to be seen by or followed up by a specialist. In the community targets can be set for establishing asthma registers within general practice and for setting up systems for regular structured review of patients by properly trained health professionals. Urgent research is also needed to identify why the condition is increasing in prevalence.

BRIAN D W HARRISON

West Norwich Hospital,
Norwich NR2 3TU

MARTYN R PARTRIDGE

Whipps Cross Hospital,
London E11 1NR

1 Burney PGJ. Strategy for asthma. *BMJ* 1991;**303**:571-3. (7 September.)
2 British Thoracic Association. Death from asthma in two regions of England. *BMJ* 1982;**285**:1251-5.
3 Bucknall CE, Robertson C, Moran F, Stevenson RD. Differences in hospital asthma management. *Lancet* 1988;i: 748-50.
4 Lorentzson S, Boe J, Eriksson G, Persson G. Use of inhaled corticosteroids in patients with mild asthma. *Thorax* 1990;**45**: 733-5.
5 Brown JP, Greville W, Finucane RE. Asthma and irreversible airflow obstruction. *Thorax* 1984;**39**:131-6.

6 Haahtelc T, Jarvinen M, Kava T. Comparison of a β_2 agonist, terbutaline, with an inhaled corticosteroid, budesonide, in newly detected asthma. *N Engl J Med* 1991;**325**:388-92.
7 Speight ANP, Lee DA, Hey DN. Underdiagnosis and undertreatment of asthma in childhood. *BMJ* 1983;**286**:1253-6.
8 Warner JO, Gotz M, Landau LI. Management of asthma: a consensus statement. *Arch Dis Child* 1989;**64**:1065-79.
9 British Thoracic Society, Research Unit of Royal College of Physicians of London, King's Fund Centre, National Asthma Campaign. Guidelines for management of asthma in adults. I: chronic persistent asthma. *BMJ* 1990;**301**:651-3.
10 British Thoracic Society, Research Unit of Royal College of Physicians of London, King's Fund Centre, National Asthma Campaign. Guidelines for management of asthma in adults. II: acute severe asthma. *BMJ* 1990;**301**:797-800.

SIR,—Professor John Garrow has produced a concise and topical summary of obesity.[1] Though I fully support his suggestion that one of the three important measures to prevent obesity should be education and the early detection of obesity at primary school age, I believe that it is important that appropriate target figures for the population in question are chosen for limiting excessive weight gain in children. In the United Kingdom an average (50th centile) child will, between 7 and 12 years, gain about 14 kg (boy) to 17 kg (girl),[2] not 22 kg as Professor Garrow states. Therefore, the suggestion that if a child gains only 18 kg over this period his or her weight will normalise is clearly not correct for British children. Indeed, this rate of weight gain for a child whose weight is on the 90th centile of weight for height will virtually maintain the centile weight for height position.

Despite recommendations to the contrary[3] weight for height centile tables are rarely used to assess obesity in British paediatric practice, though simple visual comparison of the relative centile positions of a child's weight and height on charts appropriate for the local population is commonly used. Alternative techniques to assess obesity, such as estimations of skinfold thickness, require skill in their use, the application of which is limited by interobserver error. Body mass indices with exponents specific for sex and age[4] or measurement of actual body composition by means of innovative techniques with lower interobserver error, such as bioelectrical impedance,[5] may in future prove to be of value in assessing obesity in childhood populations.

J W GREGORY

Department of Child Health,
University of Newcastle upon Tyne Medical School,
Newcastle upon Tyne NE2 4HH

1 Garrow J. Importance of obesity. *BMJ* 1991;**303**:704-6. (21 September.)
2 Tanner JM, Whitehouse RH, Takaishi M. Standards from birth to maturity for height, weight, height velocity and weight velocity: British children, 1965. Part II. *Arch Dis Child* 1966;**41**:613-35.
3 Royal College of Physicians. Obesity: a report. *J R Coll Physicians Lond* 1983;**17**:5-65.
4 Fung KP, Lee J, Lau SP, Chow OKW, Wong TW, Davis DP. Properties and clinical implications of body mass indices. *Arch Dis Child* 1990;**65**:516-9.
5 Gregory JW, Greene SA, Scrimgeour CM, Rennie MJ. Body water measurement in growth disorders: a comparison of bioelectrical impedance and skinfold thickness techniques with isotope dilution. *Arch Dis Child* 1991;**66**:220-2.

Author's reply,—I am grateful to Dr Gregory for pointing out my error concerning the normal weight gain of children: the text should have read age 5 years, not 7 years. The weights of children on the 50th and 90th centiles at age 5 years are about 18 and 22 kg and at age 12 years 40 and 54 kg, respectively. Thus the overweight child is only 4 kg overweight at age 5 and, if he or she gains 18 kg (instead of 22 kg) in the next seven years, should achieve normal weight for height.

I agree that weight for height is not an ideal measure of obesity in children, especially around puberty, when weight and height increase at different rates, but body mass index serves quite well in prepubertal children and is minimum at about age 5.[1] Bioelectric impedance is easy to measure, but most of the correlation between impedance and fat free mass is derived from the measures of weight, height, and age that are used in the prediction formulas.[2] Although impedance is claimed to measure body water, it does not accurately predict changes in body water during diuresis[3] or dialysis.[4]

JOHN GARROW

Rank Department of Human Nutrition,
St Bartholomew's Hospital Medical College,
London EC1M 6BQ

1 Rolland-Cachera MF, Cole TJ, Sempe M, Tichet J, Rossignol C, Charraud A. Body mass index variations: centiles from birth to 87 years. *Eur J Clin Nutr* 1991;45: 13-21.
2 Diaz EO, Villar J, Immink M, Gonzales T. Bioimpedance or anthropometry? *Eur J Clin Nutr* 1989;43:129-37.
3 Deurenberg P, van der Kooy K, Leenen R, Schouten FJM. Body composition changes assessed by bioelectric impedance measurements. *Eur J Clin Nutr* 1989;43:845-53.
4 De Lorenzo A, Barra PFA, Sasso GF, Battistini NC, Deurenber P. Body impedance measurements during dialysis. *Eur J Clin Nutr* 1991;45:321-5.

Sir,—Peter Anderson concludes that a strategy to reduce disease related to alcohol should have two strands: a high risk approach directed at heavy drinkers and a population approach to reduce overall consumption.[1] We agree that it would be desirable to truncate the distribution of risk by eliminating the "high tail" but share his concern that this may be difficult to achieve. Though normal distributions of physiological and behavioural variables have been moved to the left or right, we are unaware of an intervention that has altered the shape of a distribution.

Before a population strategy is adopted the costs and benefits must be weighed. Consideration should be given to the evidence that light drinkers (1-15 units a week) have a lower mortality than abstainers and occasional drinkers and that this is not entirely due to sick people stopping drinking.[2,3] Therefore the possibility of a population strategy causing harm by pushing light drinkers up the left hand side of the U shaped curve must be considered. A prospective trial might establish the value of a population strategy, but, given the difficulties of evaluating studies of dietary advice, the verdict would probably be "not proven." So apart from deploring the current lack of evidence what should the pragmatist do? We think that the association between light drinking and reduced mortality should be regarded as causal.

Strategies to reduce alcohol consumption should be examined, perhaps by mathematical modelling, and only those whose benefits outweigh the costs should be adopted.

For the present we agree with Michael Marmot and Eric Brunner that it would be inappropriate to urge people to drink more.[3] None the less, to introduce a population strategy without further analysis risks a humiliating change of policy at some future date with a subsequent loss of public confidence in advice on public health.

MICHAEL R BRADDICK

Highland Health Board,
Hilton Hospital,
Inverness IV2 3PH

CHRISTOPHER A BIRT

Highland Health Board,
Royal Northern Infirmary,
Inverness IV3 5SF

1 Anderson P. Alcohol as a key area. *BMJ* 1991;**303**:766-9. (28 September.)
2 Shaper AG, Wannamathee G, Walker M. Alcohol and mortality in British men: explaining the U shaped curve. *Lancet* 1988;ii:1267-73.
3 Marmot M, Brunner E. Alcohol and cardiovascular disease: the status of the U shaped curve. *BMJ* 1991;**303**:565-8. (7 September.)

SIR,—J M Harrington's comments on occupational health are trenchant, and many of his proposals are to be welcomed.[1] There are, however, indications that the United Kingdom is going backwards and not forwards regarding occupational health. Only a few academic departments of occupational medicine and of health and safety have ever existed, and these have recently been further reduced, "rationalised," and closed. There is also serious underfunding and understaffing of field inspectors of the Health and Safety Inspectorate and specialist support. This has paralleled a rapid growth of small and medium sized enterprises in our economy, in which occupational health staff and resources seem unlikely to be a major concern in these difficult financial times.

In the 1990s, despite the activity of a few commercial services and consultancies, there is still woefully inadequate provision of occupational health services in all but our largest companies and workplaces. At a time when markets are under close scrutiny elsewhere in the NHS and data on how they work over any length of time are lacking it is pertinent to point out the well documented failure of the marketplace to provide even basic occupational health services for many employees. Perhaps we are going back towards the sweated trade and workshop conditions of Victorian times or "on" to the South East Asian sweatshop model with all that that entails for health and safety in the workplace.

In 1941 the BMA called for "an extension of industrial medical services on both humanitarian and economic grounds" and "for more emphasis on the preventive aspects of industrial medical practice."[2] In 1991 it is surely time that the government implemented the International Labour Organisation's convention on occupational health and committed itself "to developing

233

progressively occupational health services for all workers . . . in all branches of economic activity and all undertakings."[3] The establishment of a comprehensive national occupational health service, so long advocated by some occupational physicians, is required. Such a service must involve employees (as in Italy) as well as employers and health and safety professionals in its running.[4] Only when employees are directly involved in looking after their own health and working environment will we avoid the deficiencies identified, for instance, in past NHS provision of occupational health services.

ANDREW WATTERSON

Workplace Health, Safety, and
  Environment Research Group,
Department of Adult Education,
University of Southampton,
Southampton SO9 5NH

1 Harrington JM. Work related disease and injuries. *BMJ* 1991;**303**:908-10. (12 October.)
2 The new era in industrial medicine [editorial]. *BMJ* 1943;i: 164-5.
3 Harrington JM, Gill FS. *Occupational health*. 2nd ed. Oxford: Blackwell Scientific, 1987:20.
4 Bagnara S, Misiti R, Wintersberger H, eds. *Work and health in the 1980s*. Berlin: Sigma, 1985.

SIR,—The series of articles in response to the *Health of the Nation* contains an interesting anomaly. In these statistical times it has become fashionable to describe the burden of a disease in terms of years of life lost—a measure that attempts to take account of the age at death as well as the fact of death itself—such that a death of a young person yields a higher score than a death of an older person.

There are, however, problems with such a measure. In one article in the series cancer is said to account for more years of life lost than anything else,[1] and in another accidents are said to account for a greater proportion of years of potential life lost than cancer and heart disease combined.[2] Yet another

TABLE I—Number of deaths from cancer, accidents, and coronary heart disease in district in 1990

Age band (years)	Cancer	Accidents	Coronary heart disease
0-	1	4	
15-	1	14	
25-	3	8	
35-	17	8	5
45-	53	2	19
55-	95	6	77
65-	151	4	131
≥75	244	4	344

TABLE II—Number of years of life lost depending on cut off age

Cut off age (years)	Cancer	Accidents	Coronary heart disease
55	785·5	1026	182
60	1218	1209	340·5
65	2078	1419	845
70	2985·5	1632	1389
75	4628·5	1861	2576

implies (but does not state) that coronary heart disease is top of the league table.[3] Is this another manifestation of the age old phenomenon "my specialty is more important than your specialty"? Surely they cannot all be right?

In fact, it seems as though they might all be right: the anomalies may arise because different cut off points are used. Table I shows the number of deaths from cancer, accidents, and coronary heart disease in our district in 1990. From these figures the number of years of life lost can be calculated for different cut off ages (table II). Thus with a cut off of 75 years the rank order is cancer, coronary heart disease, and then accidents. At a cut off of 65 the order is cancer, accidents, and then coronary heart disease, while at 55 the order changes yet again to accidents, cancer, and then coronary heart disease. As table II shows, accidents take the lead at a cut off somewhere between 55 and 60 years.

Clearly it is necessary, when quoting years of life lost, to specify the cut off point that has been used.

CHRIS SINCLAIR
DAVID PINDER

Department of Public Health Medicine,
West Surrey and North East Hampshire Health Authority,
Frimley,
Camberley,
Surrey GU16 5QF

1 Williams CJ. Cancer. BMJ 1991;303:516-7. (31 August.)
2 Pless IB. Accident prevention. BMJ 1991;303:462-4. (24 August.)
3 Tunstall-Pedoe H. Coronary heart disease. BMJ 1991;303: 701-4. (21 September.)

Sir,—The recent enthusiasm for setting targets based on health outcomes is welcome and long overdue, but we should beware of getting carried away. Targets for improving the health of the nation should also include assessments of managerial activities, many of which can be objectively assessed even though they cannot be quantified (see any textbook on management by objectives). Such an approach might also help to do away with the nonsense that some crucial aspects of the public health (like AIDS and food safety) are omitted from the key areas in *The Health of the Nation* because there are thought to be no measurable indicators from which to set targets.[1]

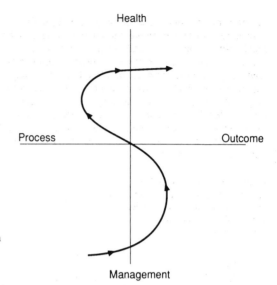

Achieving targets for
improved health
outcomes (top right
quadrant) depends
also on setting targets on
the management
processes and outcomes
that lead to them

Much of the discussion about such targets rests on a one dimensional view in which processes lead to outcomes. This traditional model has led to the current shibboleth that the only true measure of the effectiveness of health services is an outcome measure and that indicators of process are more proxies for that true measure. By this view, to assess the impact of a programme to prevent coronary artery disease you must ideally count the numbers of people with coronary artery disease—or some known risk factor—before and after the intervention of the programme. Not only are such outcomes usually slow to occur but they are fiendishly difficult and expensive to measure. It is also difficult even to obtain reliable indicators of process such as health related behaviours (for example, the proportion of the population who smoke) or the uptake of services (the numbers attending health promotion clinics).

In the figure such indicators of outcome and process would all be in the top two quadrants. But how helpful are they in indicating what action we need to take to reach targets? They cannot tell us whether the targets were reached as a result of managerial activity or despite it. The vertical axis in the figure adds this dimension to the traditional model, allowing us to distinguish whether the process and outcome are related to the people's health or to the management of the services.

After all, as the figure shows, it is managerial processes (for example, setting up an effective local task force to tackle food safety) that lead to managerial outcomes (when, for example, the task force establishes a better system for monitoring food outlets) that lead in turn to health processes (reduced consumption of unsafe foods) that lead finally to the health outcome (less food poisoning). Unless our target setting, like our audit,[2] sets out to measure our achievements in all four quadrants we shall be missing three quarters of the story and consequently less able to see where we need managerial activity to make the changes that will be necessary when—as inevitably we shall—we find we have not achieved all our health targets.

Setting clear objectives is an excellent principle when you want to achieve anything,[3] but at the risk of sounding heretical I suggest that we should not expend too much effort debating the exact level at which our health outcome targets should be set as long as they are of the right order of magnitude. It is the detailed local managerial target setting that will do most to achieve improvements in health. Thus, only by becoming closely concerned in those local managerial processes are we likely as a profession to exert our best influence on the nation's health.

JOHN GABBAY

Health Care Development Unit,
Academic Department of Public Health,
St Mary's Hospital Medical School,
Central Middlesex Hospital,
London NW10 7NS

1 Secretary of State for Health. *The health of the nation.* London: HMSO, 1991. (Cm 1523.)
2 Faculty of Public Health Medicine. *Working party report on the audit of public health medicine.* London: Faculty of Public Health Medicine, 1990.
3 Smith R. Towards a strategy for health. *BMJ* 1991;**303**:297-9. (3 August.)